2000, April 11
Erskine Mains opened by HRH Princess Anne, the Princess Royal.

2001
The Edinburgh care home opened.

2009, November 14
Edinburgh Extension – official opening by Princess Anne.

2010
Appeal launched to raise £6m to expand services.

2012, February
Erskine Print closes.

2013
Completion of rebuilding programme of 44 new cottages to meet modern energy conservation standards.

2007
Erskine Glasgow opened – official opening February 19 2008 by Princess Anne.

2000 — 2001 — 2007 — 2009 — 2010 — 2012 — 2013 — 2015 — **2016**

2012, September
Erskine Furniture closes.

2010, May
Gardening Leave who provide horticultural therapy for veterans move in to the Old Garden Centre.

2007, March
Erskine Park Home opened by Princess Anne.

2000, October 11
A new £16million, 180-bed home, which was built on the site to meet modern health criteria, was opened by Prince Charles, Erskine's patron.

1999, January
James Meechan, the last veteran from the First World War remaining at Erskine, dies aged 100.

2016, March 29
Erskine celebrates its centenary.

2015
Glasgow recreation room opens.

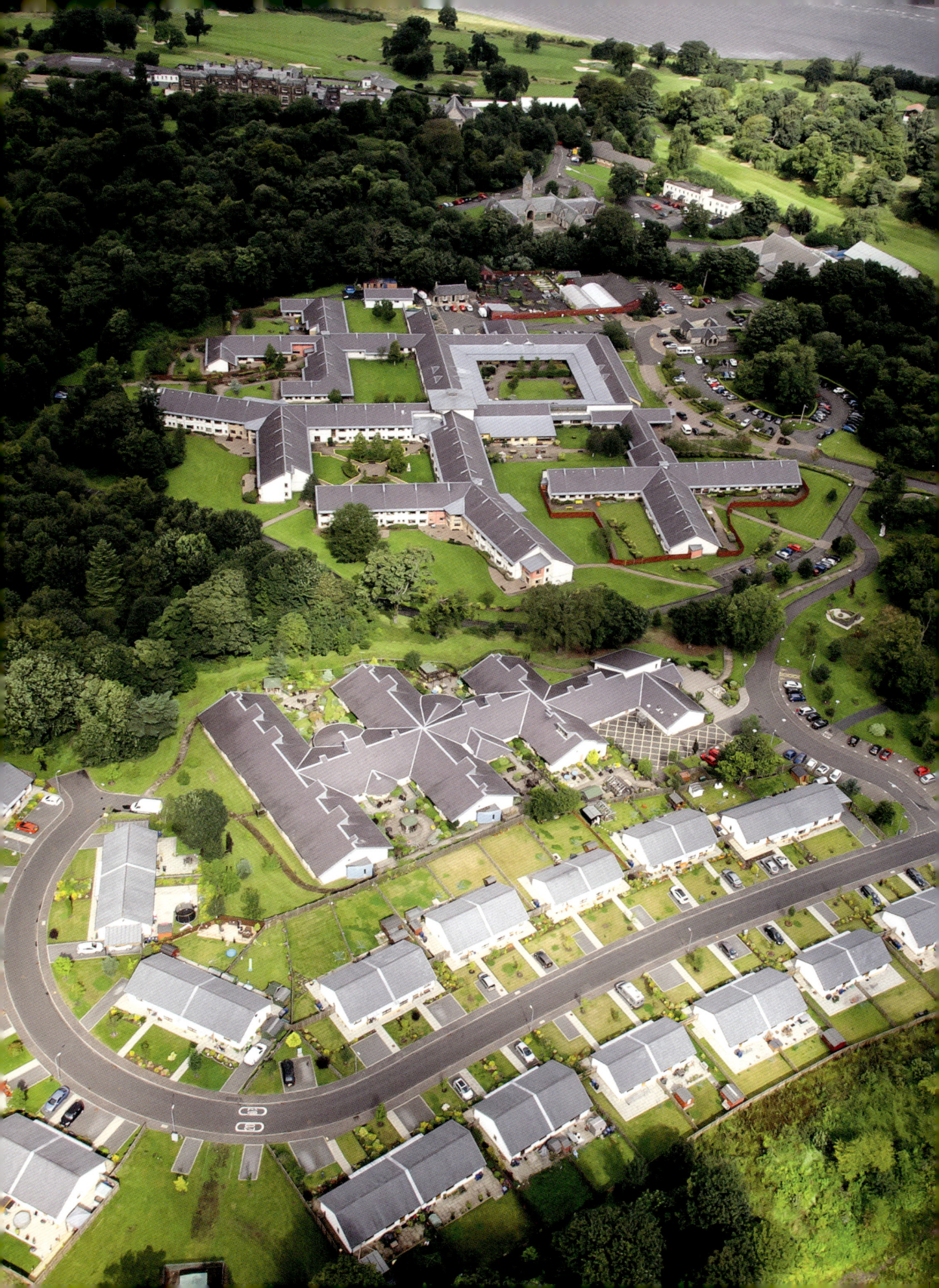

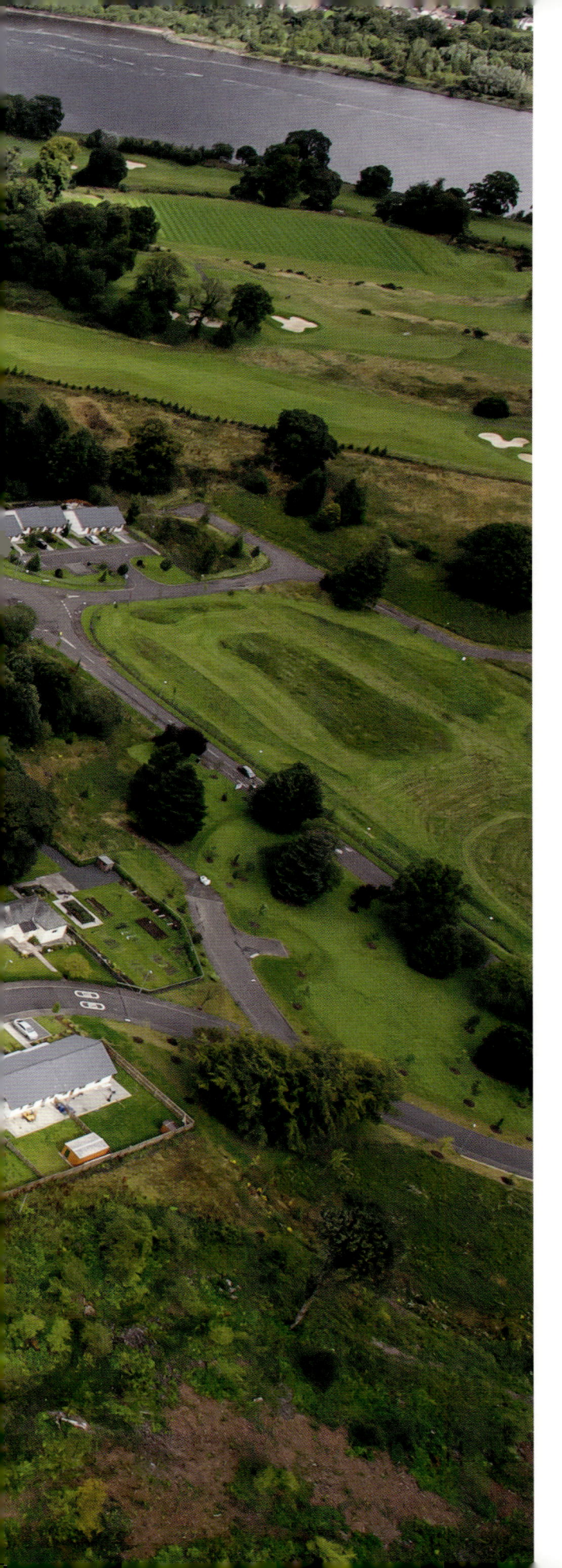

A Century Of Care: Erskine 1916–2016

AUTHORS
Anne Johnstone, Jennifer Cunningham and Russell Leadbetter

PHOTOGRAPHY
Erskine Archive

DESIGN
www.traffic-design.co.uk

WITH THANKS
This book could not have been written without the generosity of all the residents and staff and the families of former residents who gave so much time and freely shared their family albums and the personal stories which bring the Erskine spirit to life within these covers.

We are indebted also to Daniel Kelsey and Caitlyn McHarge for additional research during a project supported by Glasgow University Settlement and to Glasgow University Archives, now custodians of the Erskine records.

Susan Hamilton has been tireless in identifying interviewees and tracking down photographs. Steve Conway, Erskine's chief executive, has not only given unwavering support but provided invaluable insights.

ISBN 978-1-5262-0075-4
Published by Erskine
© 2016

Inside Cover: This impressive array of artificial limbs in a Clyde workshop in 1917, ready for use at Erskine Hospital shows the scale of the undertaking.

This page: Aerial photograph of the Erskine Home, with new houses for independent living in the foreground. The original hospital, now Mar Hall hotel can be seen beyond the trees at top left corner.

Following page: The Recreation Room at Erskine House, 1917.

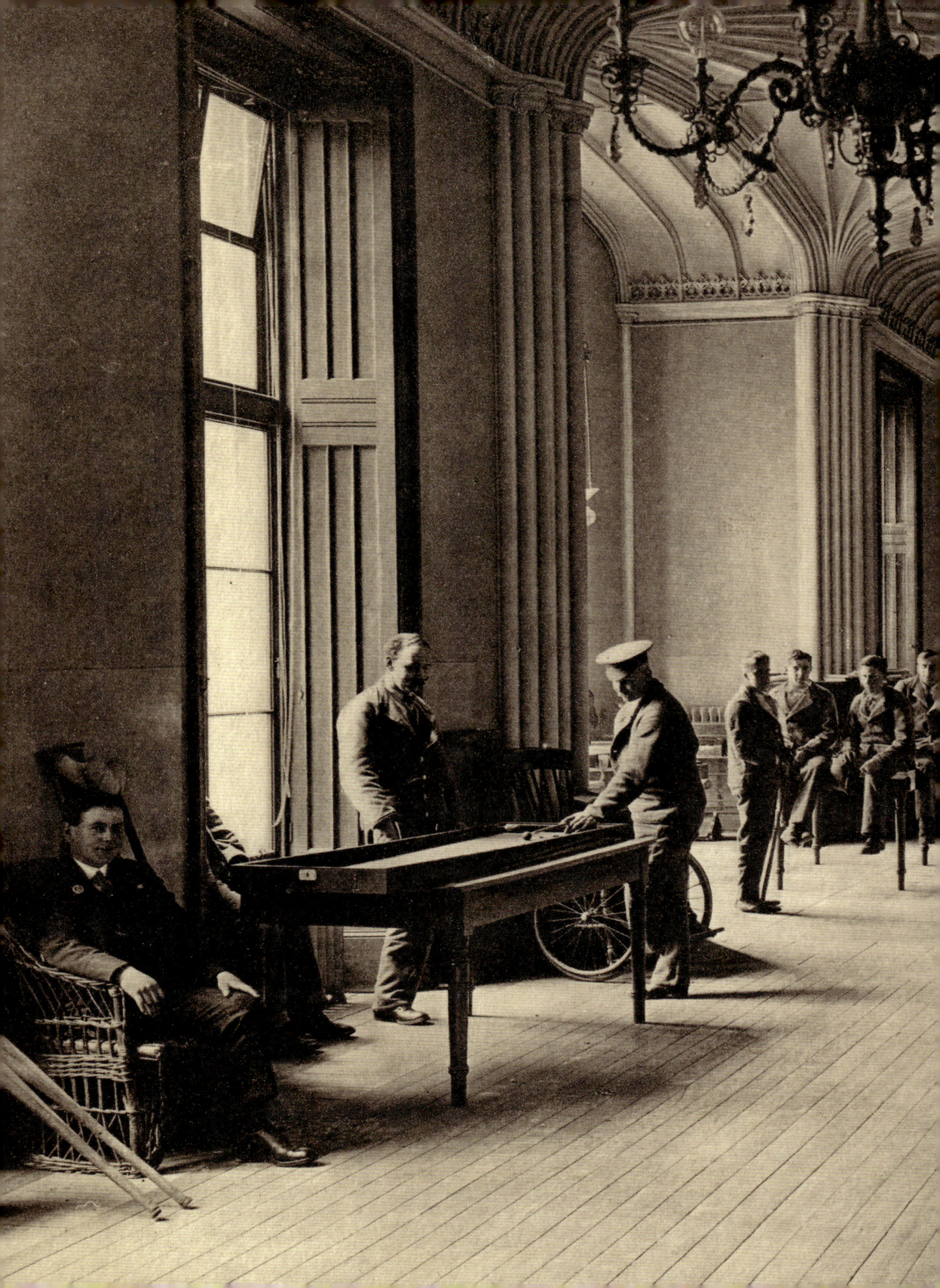

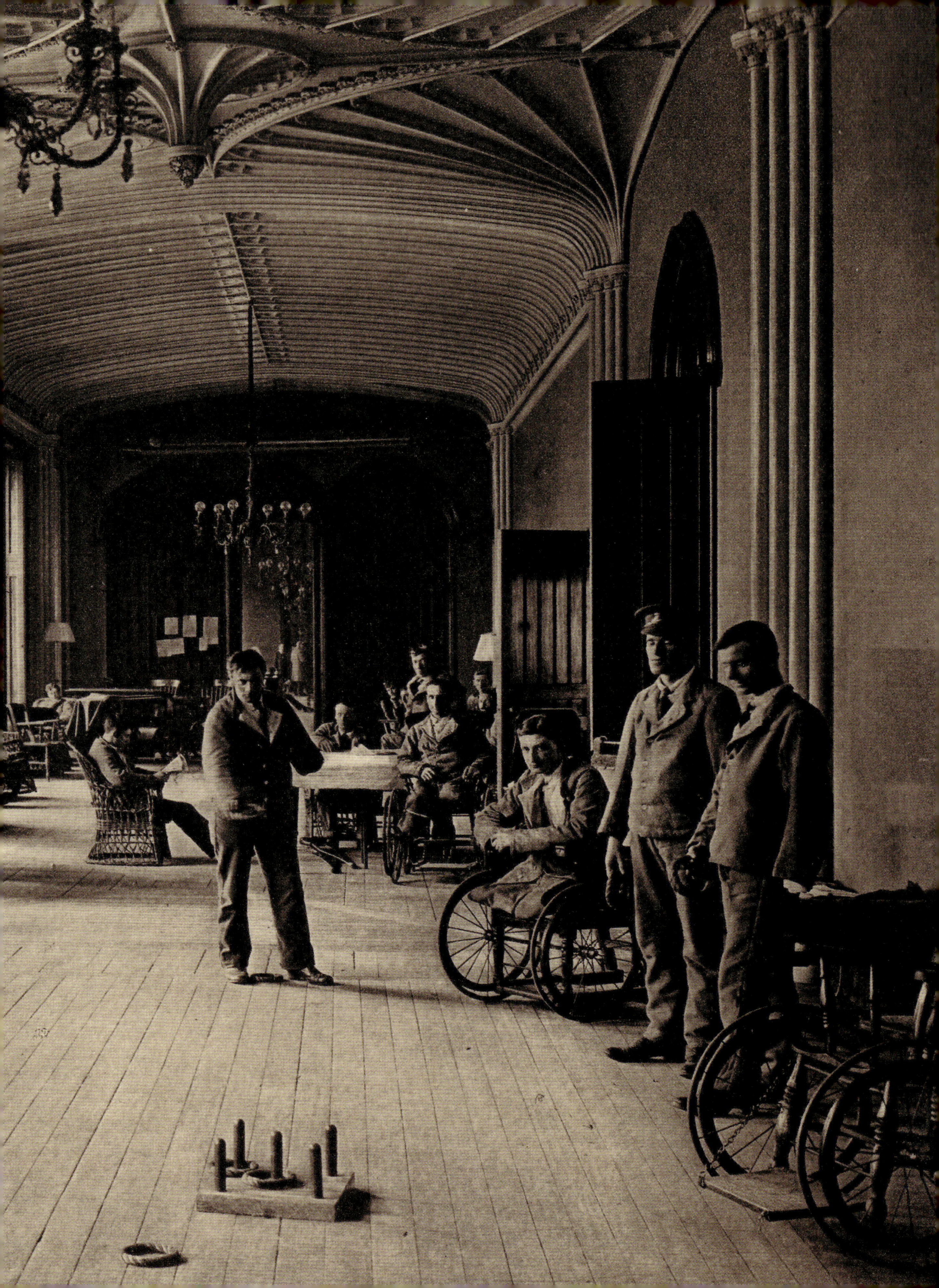

Contents

8
Foreword
by Sir Eric Yarrow

10
100 Years of Pioneering Care
How practical problem-solving and excellence in care became the hallmarks of the Princess Louise Scottish Hospital for Limbless Sailors and Soldiers.

16
Sir William Macewen
The inspiring story of the pioneering Scottish surgeon who led the project to establish the hospital and how his Erskine limb advanced the science of prosthetics.

36
Joe Parker
As aero engineer for the famed 602 Squadron (City of Glasgow), Joe Parker serviced planes for Archie McKellar, Scotland's most celebrated Spitfire ace.

40
Bill Anderson
The intriguing story of how a Navy Signalman from Maryhill played his small, vital part in history on a dockside in the Crimea.

44
Jack Harrison & Alex Lees
The amazing tale of "The Great Escape" by British Prisoners of War from Stalag Luft III in the words of two of those directly involved.

60
George Collins
The moving experience of one devastatingly-injured young soldier tackling the long road to recovery.

64
Dr Thomas McFadyen
The medical officer who regarded his patients as family and spent his spare time raising funds for additional facilities.

68
Isobel Kirkwood
How the most dedicated of Erskine's army of fundraisers, the widow of a Spitfire pilot, has raised tens of thousands of pounds for the charity.

84
From Superintendent to Commandant to Chief Executive
The men at the helm: providing leadership to meet new challenges and continuing need from 1916 to 2016.

88
Helen Bolland
Women casualties of war are relatively rare and for them specialist activities, such as sporting events for injured veterans, are invaluable.

92
John Stonham
One of today's severely injured soldiers explains their needs are the same as those of 100 years ago: understanding and a supportive environment.

22
Sir Harold Yarrow
The shipyard manager who led the manufacture of limbs and brought together the Clyde Consortium of Limb Makers.

28
James Ritson
Erskine's first official patient, awarded the DCM and Bar for gallant conduct in Gallipoli, suffered multiple bomb wounds and had his left fore-arm amputated.

32
Albert Young
An Able Seaman who took part in the Arctic Convoys, running the gauntlet of German bombers, warships and U-boats.

48
May McLean
A Glasgow girl whose long hours of work on the Bombe machines helped to break the Enigma code, tells of her experience after decades of secrecy.

52
Joe Henry
The remarkable survival of a lance corporal in the Royal Army Service Corps who was held in brutal Japanese Prisoner of War camps for over three years.

56
Maureen Lundie
Matron for 22 years, who insisted laughter was an essential ingredient of care when hospital was also home.

72
Colonel Bobby Steele
The man who executed the move of the hospital "up the road" to the new Erskine Home pays tribute to the can-do attitude of the staff.

76
Bill McDowall
The Falklands War veteran who suffered severe post-traumatic stress provides an insight into why Erskine's unique facilities are still necessary.

80
Three Generations of Caring
How five members of one family have clocked up more than a century of cleaning, caring, cooking and nursing at Erskine.

96
A New Century
How Erskine will continue to meet the challenges of providing for veterans in the twenty-first century.

100
Further Reading

Foreword
Sir Eric Yarrow MBE DL

My family's connection with Erskine goes back to the earliest days when my father joined Sir William Macewen to present the case for the original hospital at the Royal College of Surgeons in 1915, and who later became the Chairman of the Executive Committee in 1947. As a result of my parents' involvement and my own subsequent appointment as Chairman of the Executive Committee in 1980 I have been aware of the work of Erskine for much of its history, and the Yarrow family is honoured to have had such a long and close association with Erskine.

I have seen many developments over the years including the move from the original Nightingale wards in the Erskine Mansion House to single en-suite rooms in five bespoke care homes. Even in the relatively short time since their construction the Edinburgh Home has been extended and a new recreation room has been added in Glasgow to further enhance the care Erskine offers. There has also been a significant transformation in the cottages provided for veterans and their families on the Bishopton Estate, with those built after the Second World War replaced by 44 modern, energy-efficient bungalows which enable independent living.

Since the Princess Louise Scottish Hospital for Limbless Sailors and Soldiers was opened in October 1916 to treat those returning from the Western front with injuries that needed the pioneering fitting of artificial limbs, Erskine, as it is now called, has cared for over 85,000 veterans. Initially nearly all of the artificial limbs were manufactured in the pattern shop of Yarrow and Company, shipbuilders on the Clyde, until other companies and the hospital's own workshops were able to assist to meet the demand. Today Erskine provides specialist nursing and dementia care for veterans and the spouses of those who have served in the Armed Forces.

I should like to pay tribute to the nursing and care staff, managers and trustees who, throughout its history, have ensured Erskine has provided the very highest standard of care; their powerful sense of commitment and comradeship is immediately evident, creating a family environment for all the residents. I should also like to express my great confidence in the current team under the able and experienced leadership of the Chairman, Mr Andrew Robertson and Chief Executive, Lieutenant Colonel Steve Conway.

This book charts that century of care through the stories of the people of Erskine: those whose foresight and determination led to its establishment 100 years ago, veterans and their families, staff past and present and the fundraisers who maintain the unbroken tradition of generous public support that is essential to the continuation of the charity.

I remain extremely grateful to all those who support the work of Erskine and believe this book A Century of Care: Erskine 1916–2016, which brings the remarkable history of the hospital to life, is testament to that support.

Sir Eric Yarrow MBE DL

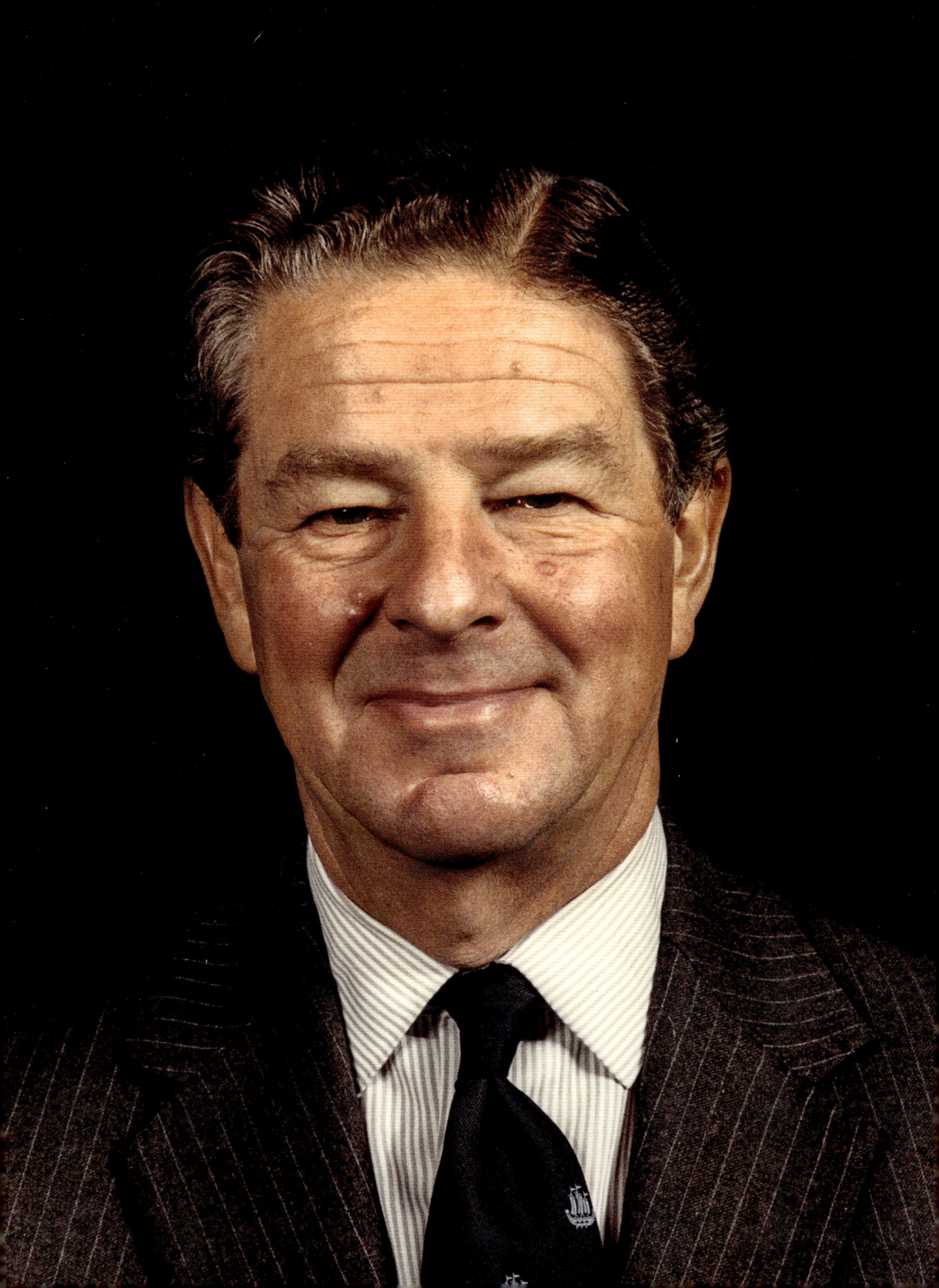

100 Years of Pioneering Care

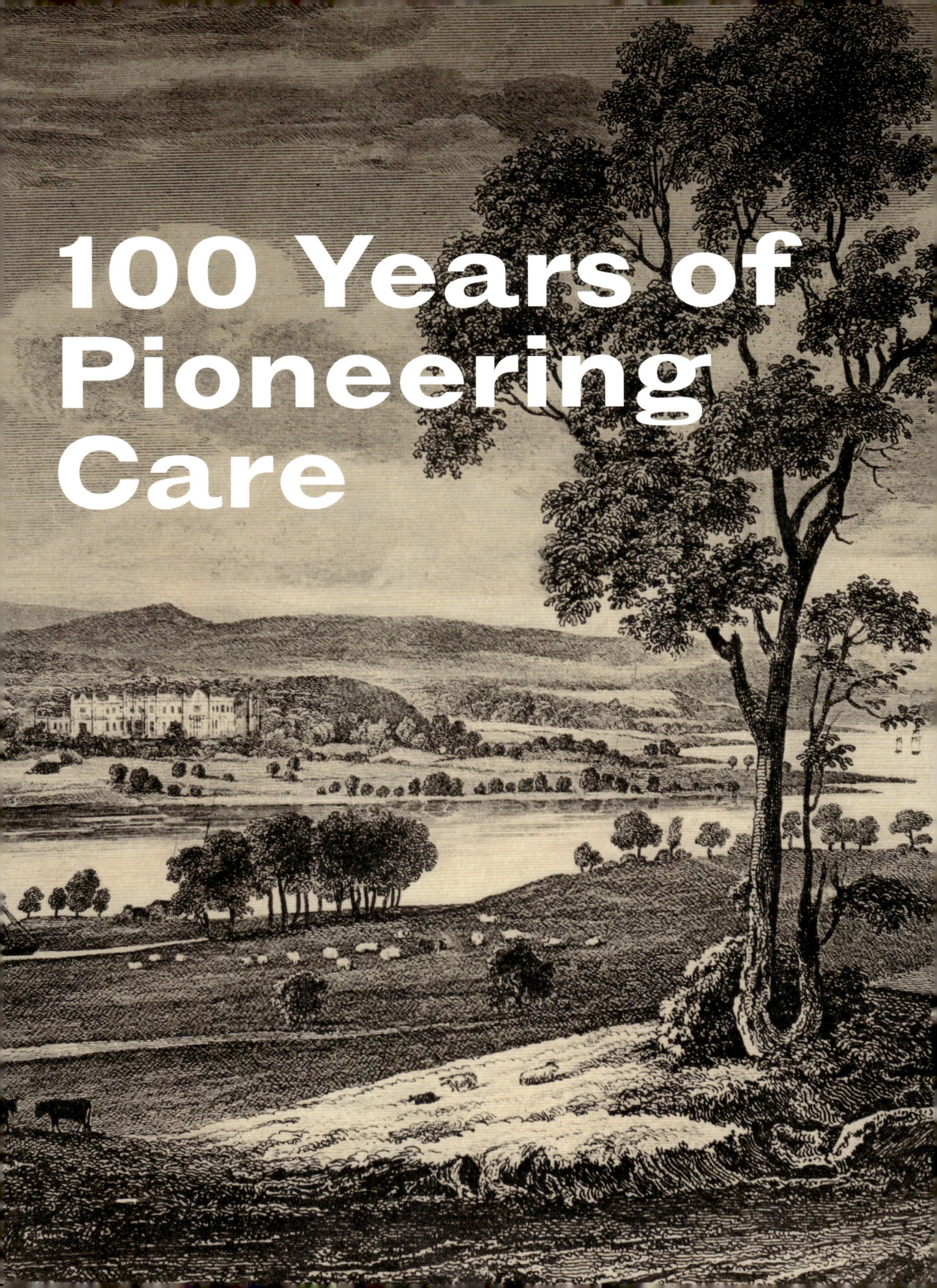

The *Princess Louise Scottish Hospital for Limbless Sailors and Soldiers* remains a unique example of mobilising expertise, finance and public support to meet an unprecedented need. The story of the institution set up by the people of Scotland to care for their wounded soldiers is as inspiring today as when the doors of Erskine House were opened to welcome those maimed on the battlefield 100 years ago. This centenary publication records the spirit of Erskine through its people from the founders, patients, doctors and nurses over the years to the residents, staff and fundraisers of today.

As the carnage from the First World War battlegrounds mounted into tens of thousands, the number of survivors who had lost limbs overwhelmed the only two hospitals specialising in the treatment of amputees, Roehampton in London and Edenhall in Musselburgh. By the autumn of 1915, there were 2000 limbless patients with nowhere to go.

In Scotland, **Sir William Macewen**, the professor of surgery at Glasgow University with a world-wide reputation for advancing surgical procedures, was appointed to lead the project to establish a new hospital dedicated to treating those whose limbs had been disastrously wounded on the battlefield.

He was the perfect choice. His pioneering operations had provided him with considerable experience in tackling the seemingly impossible, undaunted by negative perceptions of others. His reputation, fearlessness and foresight inspired others to rally to the cause. Astutely, he assembled a powerful band of fellow surgeons and those in positions of influence, such as Glasgow's Lord Provost Sir Thomas Dunlop and the principal of Glasgow University Sir Donald MacAlister, along with wealthy, well-connected individuals who aided the cause with money and expertise.

The location of the hospital was due to the generous offer by Thomson Aikman of the free use of Erskine House and its grounds at Bishopton on the south bank of the Clyde for the duration of the war and 12 months afterwards. Even more generously, Sir John Reid later provided the funds to take up Aikman's offer to sell the mansion house to the hospital if it were to become a permanent institution.

Among those invited to the initial meeting at the College of Surgeons in Glasgow in the autumn of 1915 were the engineer Professor Archibald Barr and **Harold Yarrow**, manager of the family shipyard at Scotstoun.

They proved stalwart supporters of the hospital, even as both lost sons at Ypres. As members of the limbs and appliances sub-committee they harnessed the skills of their

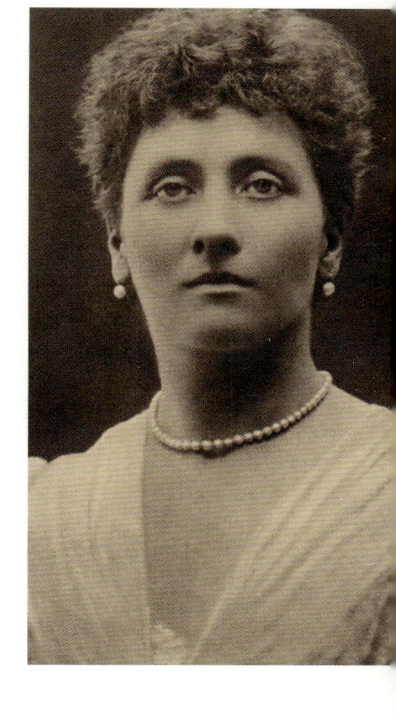

Erskine's first royal patron: Princess Louise, Duchess of Argyll.

Left: The view across the River Clyde to Erskine House. Taken from Ramsay's Views of Renfrewhire, 1939.

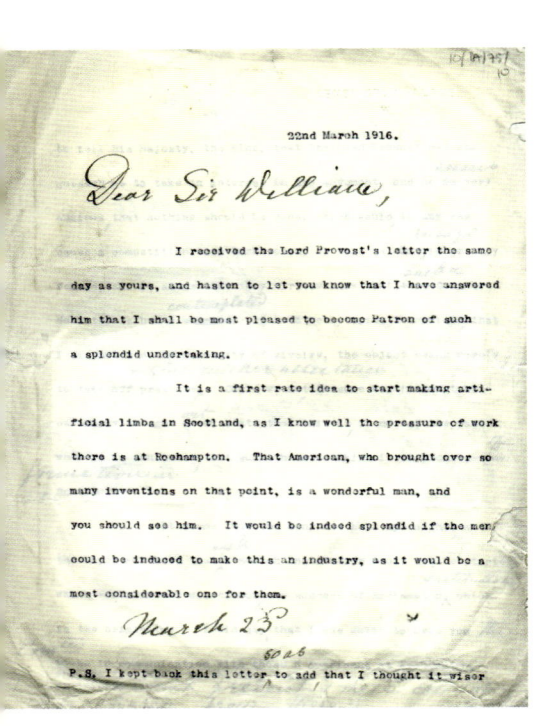

A letter from Princess Louise to Sir William Macewen on March 22, 1916, confirming her patronage of the "first rate idea."

renowned workforces to the production of artificial limbs. These and the other yards which made up the Clyde Consortium of Limbs Makers more than justified Sir William Macewen's confidence. It was his determination that those who suffered amputation of their limbs should be provided with an artificial limb which would function as well as possible, that resulted in the Erskine Provisional Limbs setting a new standard in prosthetics. Described as masterpieces of lightness and simplicity, the prototypes took various forms. The simplest little more than a broomstick fixed to a disc of wood, while others had knee joints or a simple foot but each was carefully fitted and capable of adjustment with straps where it was fitted to the stump with a "bucket" of thin, pliable wood. With experience and continued research, and the help the best engineers and craftsmen lent by the Clyde yards, improvements evolved to make them lighter than other limbs of the time without sacrificing strength.

The records of the shipbuilder, Stephen of Linthouse, provide an insight into how the yards took up this new challenge. "In addition to supplying armaments, Linthouse also undertook the manufacture of artificial feet and ankles, under the direction of Yarrows. These limbs, which were made in the modelmakers' shop, from rough beechwood blocks to several sizes, proved highly satisfactory when completed with fittings and polished. As the shop was of moderate size, the workers were limited to one foreman and nine joiners; despite its small staff this detachment completed and delivered 2175 feet and ankles between April, 1917 and June, 1920."

The first patients were received at Erskine House in October 1916, with **James Ritson** from Troon appearing first on the register. The formal opening ceremony was performed by the hospital's patron, Her Royal Highness Princess Louise, on June 6, 1917.

By 1924, 8000 of the 41,000 permanently disabled veterans in Britain had been treated at Erskine, with 6400 supplied with artificial limbs. It was a truly extraordinary feat but the real measure of success was that the majority, fitted with new arms or legs, having mastered new ways of walking and using their arms and perhaps having learned a new trade such as bootmaking, tailoring or hairdressing, left the shelter of the hospital to resume life where they had left off. They did so with determination and courage, many managing to walk considerable distances and even play golf and bowls in defiance of their disability. The hospital's focus was already beginning to change from surgical operations and rehabilitation towards providing permanent care and supported accommodation for disabled ex-servicemen.

Five years after the end of the First World War, however, Erskine faced a new challenge when the Ministry of Pensions asked Erskine to provide beds for patients with tuberculosis resulting from war service.

Of course it rose to the challenge, despite the concerns noted by the executive committee that these patients required prolonged care and often did not recover.

Matching resources to need in the most efficient and beneficial way has been a continuous challenge for the trustees. In the mid-1920s there was already a debate over the sustainability of administration by "a multiplicity of standing committees." A new step in fundraising was taken on Christmas Day 1927 when Harold Yarrow made a broadcast appeal on behalf of the hospital.

With the outbreak of the Second World War, Erskine was expected to deal with the wounded and the long-unused huts from the First World War were refurbished to provide

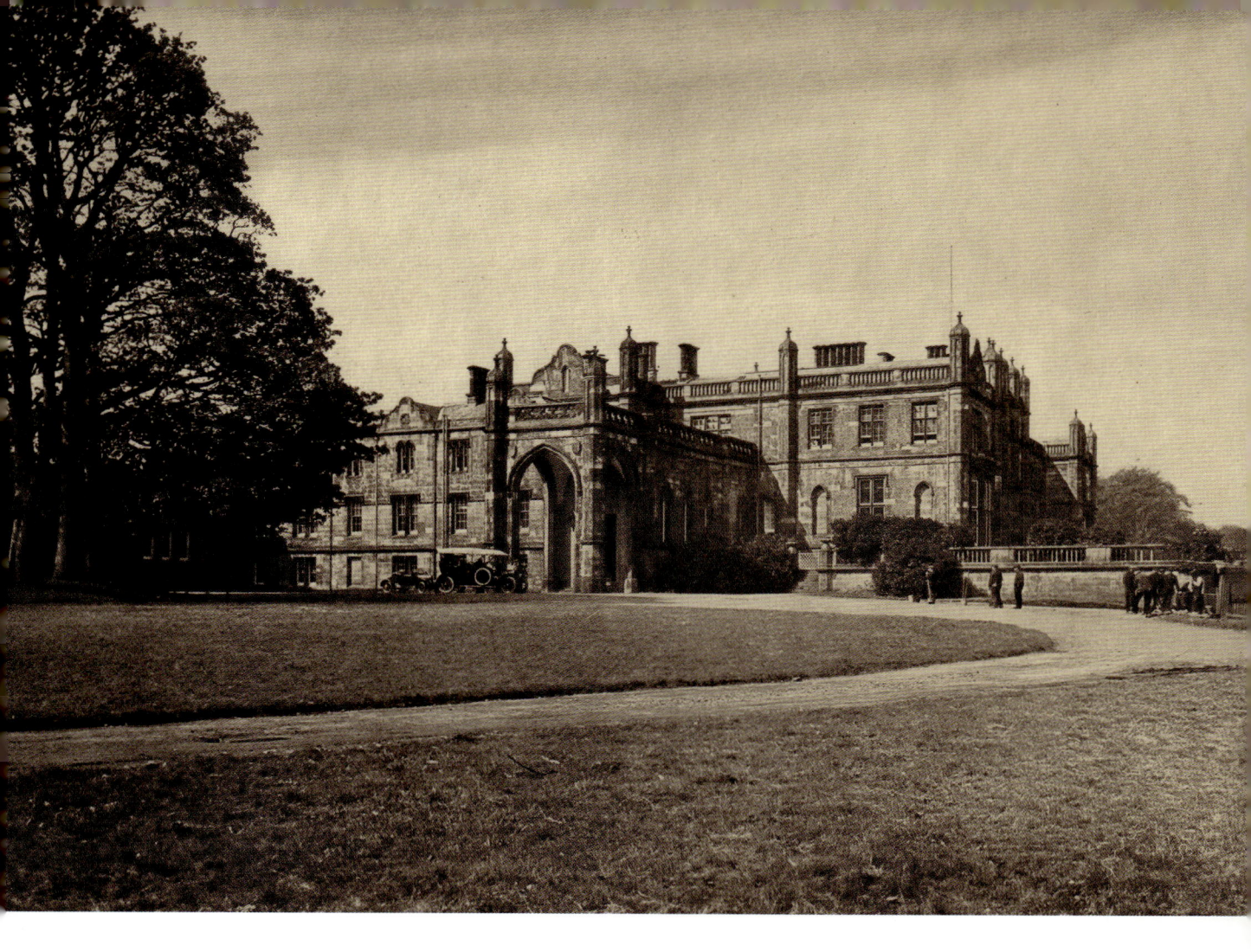

The main entrance and grounds to the hospital at Erskine House, 1917.

200 beds. In addition to casualties from the war, the hospital cared for civilians injured in the Blitz on the West of Scotland. In 1945, there were 740 patients from the Second World War in addition to 150 First World War veterans.

A new phase in what the charity could provide for veterans began with the building of cottages where war pensioners could live with their families in the grounds. These were funded by donations, including a major one from the Scottish Veterans' Garden City Association. Among the very varied residents who served in 1939-45 were some remarkable individuals. **Albert Young** sailed in the Arctic convoys in the North Atlantic and was on HMS Windsor when she was torpedoed. **Joe Parker** was RAF mechanic to celebrated Spitfire pilot, Archie McKellar. **Bill Anderson** was a Navy signalman who was able to guide Churchill and Anthony Eden, the Foreign Secretary through the darkness at the Yalta Conference. **Jack Harrison** and **Alex Lees**, prisoners of war in Germany who were involved in the plot which became known as "The Great Escape." **Joe Henry**, a prisoner of war in Japan, who brought up his family in one of the cottages at Erskine. **May McLean**, a Wren, who worked as a codebreaker.

Although new buildings, including a gym, new wards and nurses' quarters had been added by 1946, it was obvious further expansion was required. The advent of the National Health Service raised the question of whether this hospital funded by donations could remain independent. In March 1948, to the committee's delight, the Department of Health for Scotland decided the Erskine Hospital did not have to be transferred to the NHS.

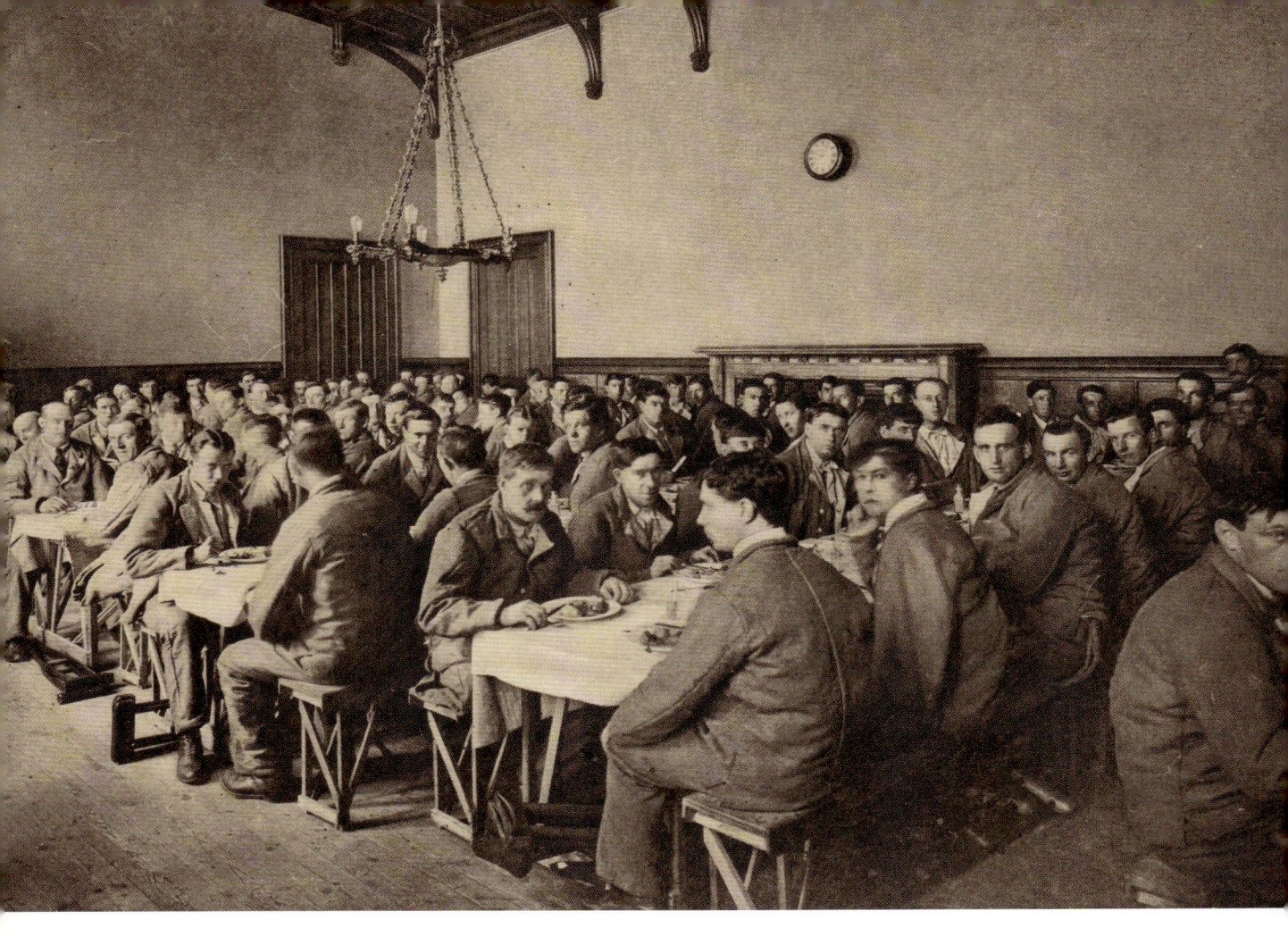

Mealtime in the hospital dining room.

A new convalescent wing funded by the Red Cross was completed in 1950 and a hostel built for men employed in the workshops. The opening of a two-storey block for acute medical and surgical cases involved a major re-organisation with patients moving into newer facilities and the ground floor of the mansion house becoming dining rooms.

In 1966, when Erskine celebrated half a century of care, it was also time for a realistic assessment of future demands. The expectation that the number of disabled veterans of the First World War would be greatly reduced, while the number of Second World War veterans being cared for by Erskine would increase, proved accurate. The role of Erskine Hospital had changed to meet the different needs of a new age. Care was no longer restricted to the limbless of 1914-18 but extended to all ex-servicemen who had become disabled, whether as a direct result of combat or from other causes.

By 1978 running costs had escalated to reach £1million a year due to a combination of inflation, a spike in the price of oil for heating and a sharp increase in nurses' wages. To make ends meet, it was necessary to liquidate some investments and take out a bank loan. At the annual meeting of the executive committee in 1978, the chairman, General Sir Gordon MacMillan, announced the Effort for Erskine fundraising scheme which highlighted the personal stories of some of the veterans and produced a generous response from the public.

Erskine would not have been able to weather this financial crisis, however, without an important change in funding arrangements. The executive committee and senior staff had always argued that Erskine, as a unique hospital for service veterans, should remain outwith the National Health Service. In pre-devolution times, the Scottish Office was sympathetic to its claim to be treated as a special case but power rested in London. Fortunately, Betty Harvie Anderson, then MP for East Renfrewshire and Deputy Speaker of the House of Commons, was a member of Erskine's executive committee. As the daughter of one of the hospital's founders, Colonel Thomas Harvie Anderson, and someone who had seen service on the Home Front as a member of the ATS during the Second World War, she was a feisty supporter of Erskine.

Her pleading of the cause along with Harry Ewing, then Scottish health minister, resulted in an announcement that the government would bear the cost of every war pensioner undergoing treatment for his pensionable disability at Erskine plus an additional 30 ex-service patients who would otherwise have to be treated by the NHS.

This was a vital intervention at a time when Erskine had to use about £100,000 of its capital reserves for running costs. Once again, the generosity of the public exceeded expectations, with the treasurer able to report at the end of the year that donations had reached a peak level of £336,055.

The tradition of financial support for Erskine from fundraising events and the generosity of individuals has continued throughout its entire history. Few, however, are as dedicated as **Isobel Kirkwood**. Fundraising has become the focus of her life in gratitude for the care provided to her husband a former RAF Spitfire pilot who was later disabled by multiple sclerosis.

By the 1990s with better services for disabled people in the NHS and by other charities the original concept of the hospital had changed.

Over the decades since the two world wars, because Erskine had been caring for those wounded veterans who would never be able to find a way of coping in mainstream society, it gradually became an elderly care provider. Its original purpose continues, nevertheless, in providing care and accommodation for younger people injured in more recent conflicts. Among those living in cottages on the Erskine estate are **George Collins**, who was very seriously injured in Northern Ireland, **Bill McDowall**, who was injured in The Falklands and is now Erskine's IT manager, **Helen Bolland**, who served with the RAF in Iraq and **John Stonham** who sustained horrific injuries in Iraq.

As Erskine's main task became providing elderly care, rather than hospital treatment, it became increasingly clear that the mansion house was no longer fit for purpose. Its fate was sealed when new regulations for care homes were introduced in 1993. It was an ambitious undertaking to build brand new facilities but, once again, the public responded magnificently.

The mansion house, which had done sterling service for 75 years was sold to become the five-star Mar Hall Hotel, named for the Earls of Mar, originally granted the Erskine lands by King Malcolm II.

The Erskine 2000 initiative included building the Erskine Home, for 180 residents, which was opened on the Bishopton estate in 2000, a second new home, Erskine Mains, in the town of Erskine, where the 34 residents would be closer to all the facilities and Erskine Edinburgh, which was opened in 2002 and provides nursing and dementia care for 88 residents. As we shall see later, there is a commitment to continue to meet the needs of injured service personnel who receive medical treatment from the NHS but require accommodation and support to make a full recovery.

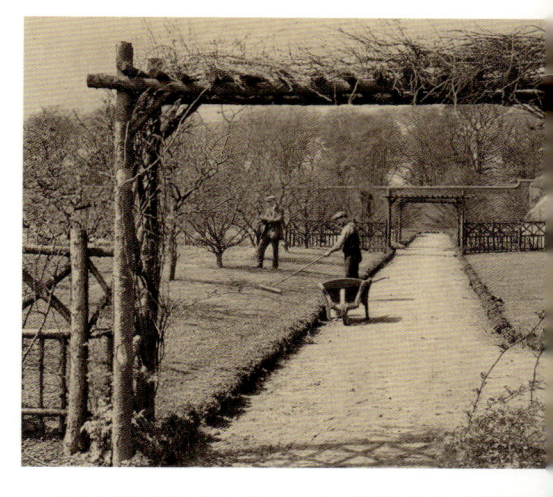

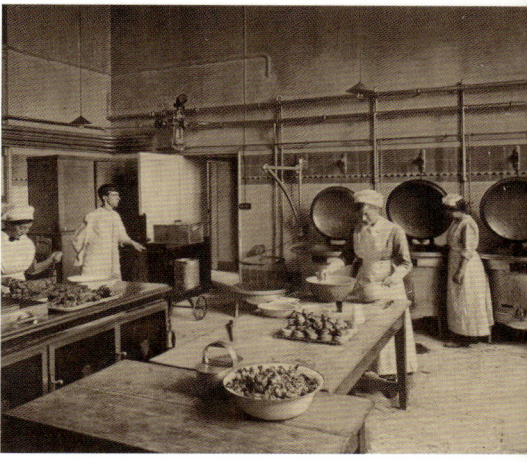

Top: the garden grounds at Erskine House provided space for exercising new limbs.

Above: Kitchen staff prepare a meal for the patients.

Sir William Macewen

"To obtain the best results, sympathetic care and encouragement are required, besides advice and guidance. That is what is aimed at in the auxiliary hospital proposed."

Without Sir William Macewen, the Princess Louise Scottish Hospital for Limbless Sailors and Soldiers would not have been the pioneering establishment which led the world in the design, manufacture and fitting of artificial limbs. It was his formidable leadership which galvanised support across all sections of society and drove the project to convert Erskine House, which was ready to receive the first patients just over six months later.

At over six feet in height, he was a big man in every sense. In 1915 when the need for a new specialist hospital in Scotland to treat the overwhelming flow of casualties from the front had become a matter of urgency, he was world-renowned for his advances in surgery (later acknowledged as 50 years ahead of his time) with a string of international honours. He was also Regius Professor of Surgery at the University of Glasgow and seen as the man most likely to be effective in setting up a new hospital from scratch. He received unanimous backing for the project at a meeting of Glasgow's senior surgeons and quickly formed a provisional committee, immediately co-opting people of influence outwith the medical profession, including wealthy landowners and industrialists, such as Harold Yarrow. They were to play key roles in the project, providing financial support and the engineering skills which were to make the Erskine venture so much more than a hospital.

Macewen's own broad range of skills and a compassion for his patients that extended to their wellbeing beyond the physical treatment of their disabilities laid the foundation for the ethos of caring for every individual as a person rather than a patient that continues to this day.

Born in 1848 at Woodend, close to Rothesay on Bute, his island childhood gave him a lifelong love of nature and sailing. Importantly for the medical advances he was to make, and for Erskine, it also provided opportunities for gaining manual skills such as building model boats and triggered an insatiable curiosity about how things worked. He learned early that the answers could be found by careful observation. Thus after studying how damaged antlers on deer could repair themselves, he was convinced that the teaching of the time was wrong and experimented with new ways of bone-grafting. His method became standard practice.

His medical career was impressive from the beginning. He graduated from Glasgow University at the age of 21 and became a consultant surgeon at 25. His ability to combine new, scientific understanding with technical precision enabled him to operate where others feared it would be fatal to insert a scalpel. It is difficult for us to contemplate surgery to remove brain tumours at a time before the X-ray was discovered, yet for Macewen, close observation of a patient's impairment would provide the key to establishing which part of the brain was affected.

The surgical advances he made are key to understanding the pioneering approach he

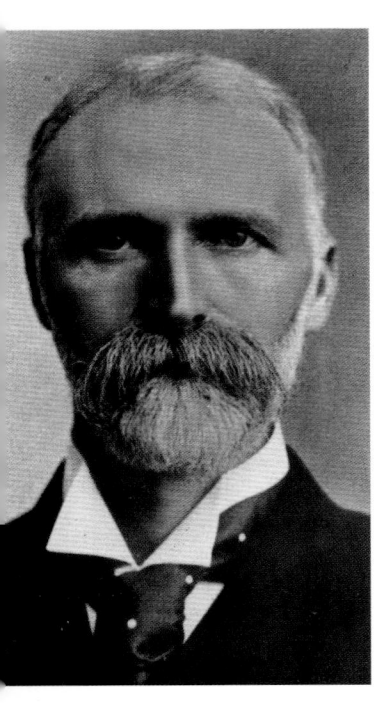

Above: Sir William Macewen, pioneering surgeon and the driving force in establishing the hospital.

Right: Minutes from the public meeting at Glasgow City Chambers where Sir William Macewen addressed the urgent need for a specialist hospital in Scotland.

PRINCESS LOUISE SCOTTISH HOSPITAL FOR LIMBLESS SAILORS AND SOLDIERS.

MINUTES OF MEETINGS.

At GLASGOW, and within the Council Hall of the City Chambers there, on Wednesday, 29th March, 1916. — 29th March, 1916.

Met the Right Honourable the LORD PROVOST OF GLASGOW (Thomas Dunlop, Esq.), and many Citizens of Glasgow and the West of Scotland, for the purpose of hearing Statements as to the objects and scope of a Proposed Hospital for Maimed and Limbless Sailors and Soldiers in the West of Scotland. — *Public meeting of Citizens of Glasgow and the West of Scotland.*

Among many others present were:—The Marchioness of AILSA, Lord and Lady INVERCLYDE, Lord NEWLANDS, Sir THOMAS GLEN-COATS, Bart.; Sir JAMES BELL, Bart.; Sir WILLIAM and Lady MACEWEN, Sir ARCHIBALD M'INNES SHAW, Mrs. T. DUNLOP, Dr. JAMES A. ADAMS, Mr. J. H. PRINGLE, Mr. R. A. OSWALD of Auchencruive, Mr. THOMSON AIKMAN of Erskine, Professor and Mrs. BARR, Mrs. POLLOCK, Glenfairn, Ayr; Miss ANDERSON, Barskimming; Mr. and Mrs. DAVID M'COWAN, Mr. and Mrs. JOHN REID, Mr. HAROLD E. YARROW, Colonel J. SMITH PARK, M.V.O.; Mr. C. J. CLELAND, M.V.O.; Mr. and Mrs. H. CARVICK WEBSTER, Dr. J. A. C. MACEWEN and Miss MACEWEN, Mr. THOMAS BINNIE, Mr. JOHN S. SAMUEL, Mr. WILLIAM GUY.

The Right Honourable the Lord Provost presided.

The Lord Provost and Sir William Macewen gave explanatory statements as to the objects and scope of the scheme, and pleaded its claims to the generous consideration of the public. — *Explanatory statements.*

Thereafter the Lord Provost moved and Sir William Macewen seconded a resolution approving of the establishment of a hospital, to be called "The Princess Louise Scottish Hospital for Limbless Sailors and Soldiers," and commending it to the generous consideration of all interested in the welfare of the men who, after fighting for King and Country, return maimed and crippled. This resolution on being put to the meeting was carried with acclamation. — *Resolution establishing hospital.*

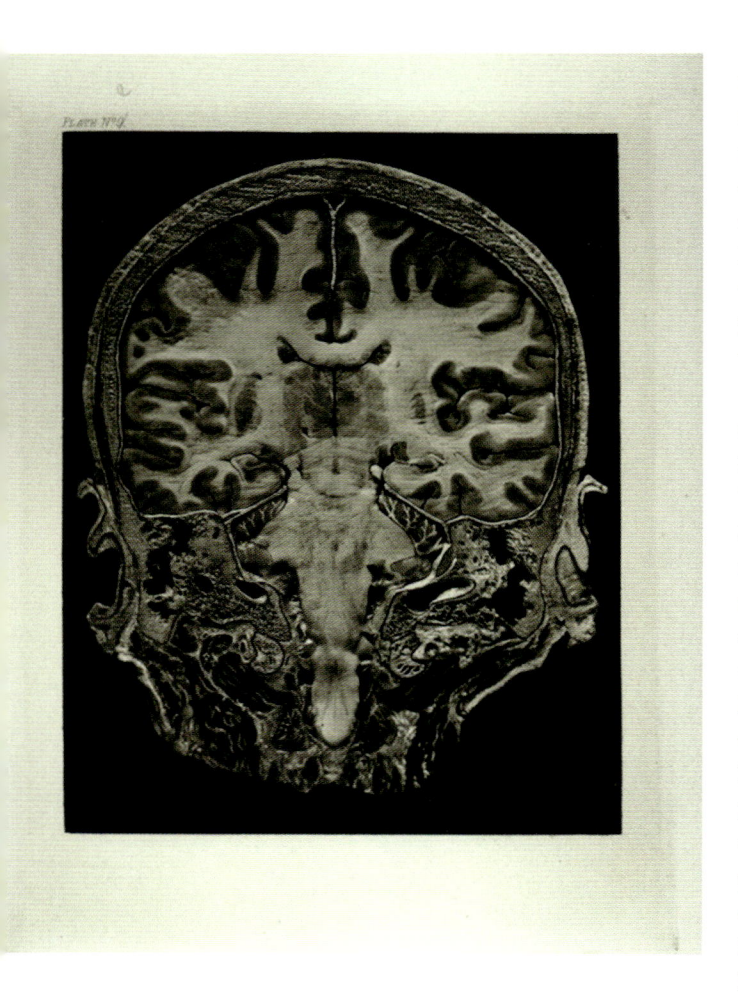

One of the copperplate engravings cut by Macewen in his Atlas of Head Sections.

took to the challenge of providing artificial limbs for amputees. He demonstrated in 1876 that it was possible to use a precise clinical examination to determine the possible site of a tumour or lesion in the brain, by observing its effects on the alterations in motor and sensory functions. He diagnosed an abscess in the frontal lobe of a boy in this way but the family refused permission to operate. When the patient died his diagnosis and site of the abscess were found to be correct.

In 1879, he was the first surgeon to remove a tumour from the brain, establishing his world-wide reputation. Nine years later, in an address on the surgery of the brain, "the most wonderful machine in the world," he told astounded members of the British Medical Association meeting in Glasgow: "Surgery of the brain has its limits but these have not been reached." This was neither self-aggrandisement nor wishful thinking. Macewen had an extraordinary success rate, prompting a US neurosurgeon, DJ Canale of the University of Tennessee, to pay tribute to the Scots pioneer in 1996. Writing in the Journal of Neurosurgery, Canale cited the importance of Macewen's paper, Pyogenic Infective Diseases of the Brain and Spinal Cord, and its accompanying volume, Atlas of Head Sections, published just over a century earlier in 1893. "Macewen's diagnosis was based on clinical findings superbly illustrated by his three clinical stages of brain abscess development. His clinical observations are as relevant today as when he described them 100 years ago Macewen recorded 25 cases of brain abscess. Nineteen of these patients came to his attention in time to undergo surgery, resulting in 18 recoveries. All five of his patients with extradural abscess recovered. These results were achieved in the era known as 'the most glorious period in British surgery'. Neurosurgery was in its infancy; nevertheless, even as the 20th century closes, Macewen's results still have not been surpassed."

The Atlas of Head Sections consisted of 53 engraved copperplates of frozen sections of the head. Each one was cut by Macewen himself. At that time, the work was at the forefront of scientific achievement and the New York Medical Herald stated that it surpassed "all others in perfection of its execution and in the completeness of the work."

In 1895, he performed the world's first successful removal of a lung, with the patient not only surviving but able to lead a normal, active life.

The success of these daring feats of surgery owed much to the fact they were always preceded by meticulous investigation. Charles Duguid, a distinguished surgeon who studied under Macewen, recalled in Macewen of Glasgow – a Recollection of the Chief, that every operation involved the most painstaking investigation and careful diagnosis: "As an operator, he was deliberate and fearless rather than fast."

The nature of such breakthrough operations was determined simply by the needs of patients. Faced with many children in Glasgow with legs deformed by rickets, he devised the operation to break and straighten the bones, which became the technique used in all industrial cities where the disease was prevalent.

It should be remembered that his astonishing success rate was not due to surgical skill alone.

He worked very closely with the matron of Glasgow Royal Infirmary, Rebecca Strong, in setting out a training programme for nurses – which would be copied throughout the world.

His work on antisepsis and progression to asepsis (the state of being free from disease-causing contaminants) was inspired by another medical pioneer, Joseph Lister, his professor and later friend.

Macewen's 1912 biography of Lister (Lord Lister) contains a description of his subject that could equally apply to himself. "He was a man in earnest and therefore he taught. He accumulated data by observation and experiment, from both of which careful deductions were drawn." It was by following Lister's prescription for deep cleansing and disinfection of hands and arms, sterilisation of surgical tools, use of surgical gowns, and the recent discovery of anaesthesia, that Macewen became able to greatly advance modern surgical technique and improve the recovery of patients.

Shortly after the outbreak of the First World War, Macewen was commissioned as Surgeon-General in Scotland for the Royal Navy, with the Rank of Surgeon Rear-Admiral. His naval work included supervising and caring for the naval and military wounded at Mount Stuart House on Bute and at Dungavel, the former hunting lodge of the Dukes of Hamilton in addition to his clinical teaching at the Western Infirmary in Glasgow.

The establishment of the Princess Louise Scottish Hospital for Limbless Sailors and Soldiers, at Erskine House, however, a cause he took up with characteristic single-mindedness, was undoubtedly his greatest legacy from the First World War. Early in 1916, Sir Donald MacAlister, principal of Glasgow University and himself a physician, was asked by the English authorities, overwhelmed by the numbers of limbless combatants, if suitable accommodation, materials and technical assistance could be provided in Scotland. He asked Macewen to become chief organiser of the scheme and received the robust response: "I'll take it up on one condition – that you do not ask other surgeons to co-operate; I am not a co-operator." The principal apparently recognised that his Professor of Surgery was a force of nature best left to take its own course. The result was extraordinary progress.

It was Macewen, of course, who, having secured the backing of his fellow surgeons, headed the deputation from the Provisional Committee of the great and good to outline the proposal for a new military hospital to the Lord Provost of Glasgow, Sir Thomas Dunlop. He gave his immediate support and convened the public meeting in the city chambers on March 29, 1916 at which Sir William Macewen's speech setting out the need for a specialist hospital dedicated to the treatment and care of amputees roused public sympathy and support to such an extent that £100,000 was contributed within a few weeks and doubled within a year.

His speech provides us with an insight into two elements at the core of this extraordinary man: a deep compassion for his fellow human beings and a "can do" approach to any challenge. He explained why specialist care was urgently needed. "After an amputated limb

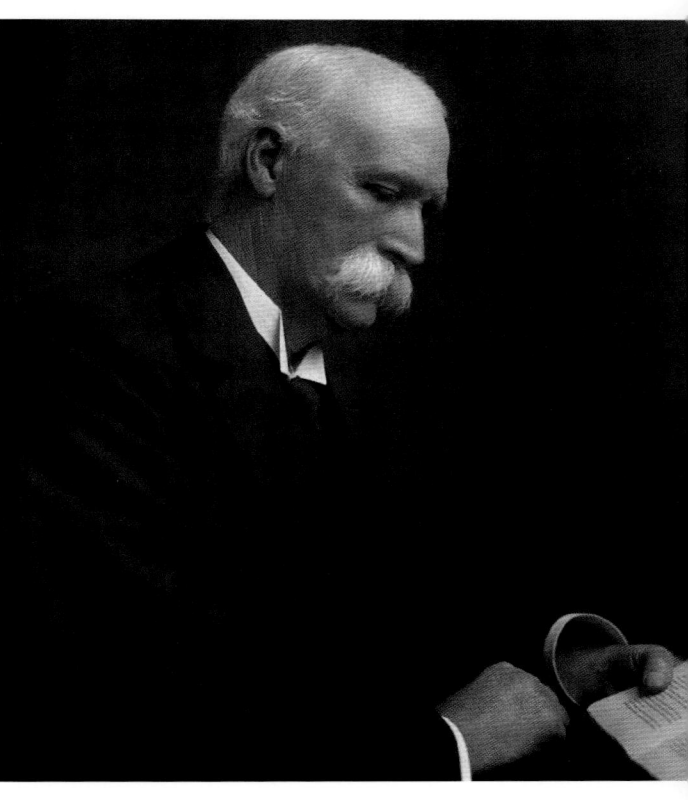

Sir William remained Regius Professor of Surgery at Glasgow University until his death in 1924 but the hospital at Erskine was his "special child."

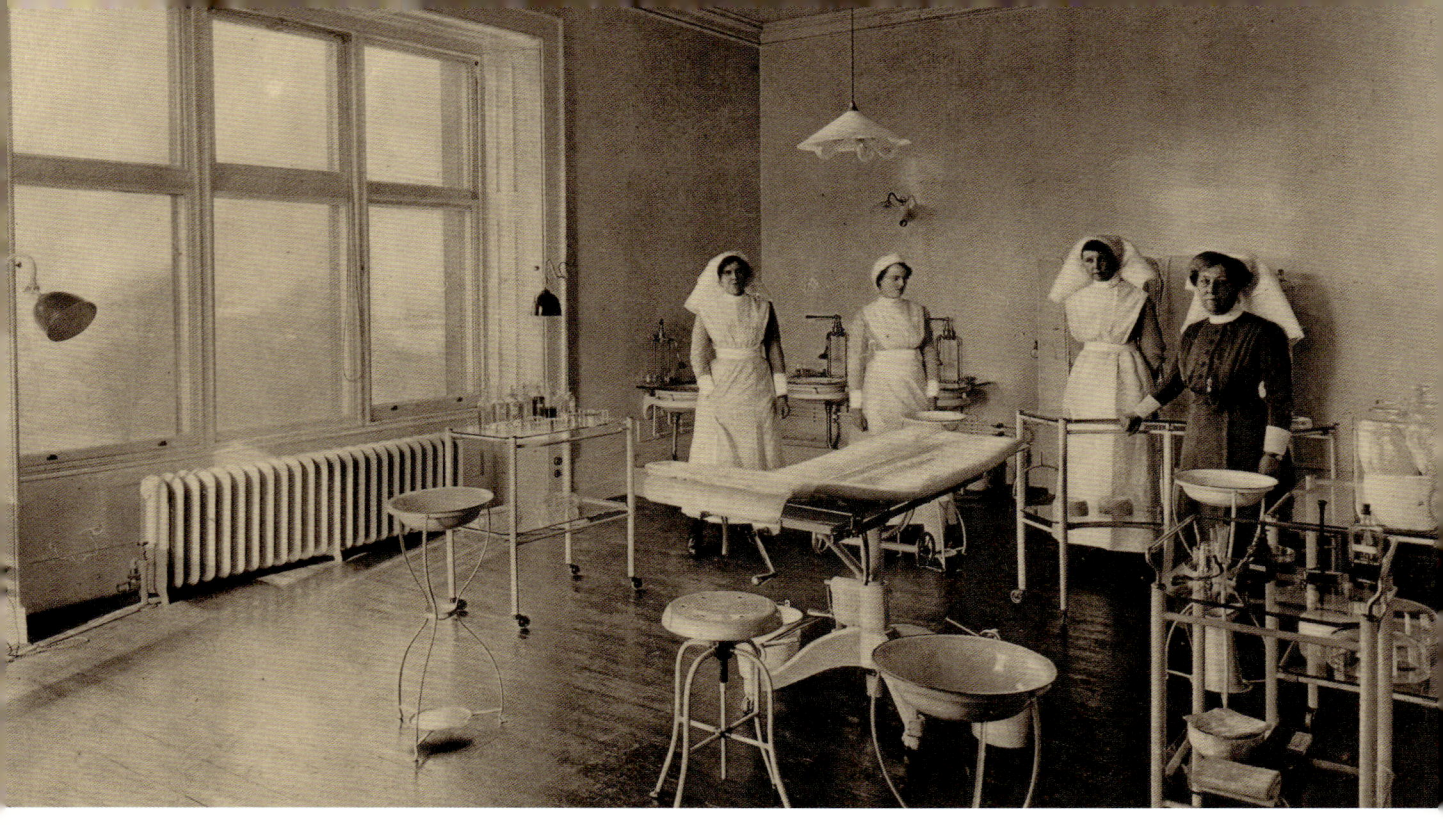

The original operating theatre in the converted mansion.

has healed, patients are sent out of the large hospitals whilst their stumps are still too tender and swollen to permit of artificial limbs being applied. Weeks and possibly months may elapse before the artificial limb can be borne, and during this period of waiting much may be done."

It was recognition once again that surgery, however vital, was part of a process, requiring other good practice such as nursing care and help to return to normal life.

He made a persuasive case for what would now be called physiotherapy and occupational therapy and the benefits of providing training to enable all who were capable to gain employment. But it was the response to his heartfelt appeal to the pride in the technical skills of Clydeside that led to the production of world-class artificial limbs and made Erskine synonymous with top quality.

His words retain a power to rival Kitchener's 1914 call to arms. They must have been electrifying in 1916. "We were told that it would be impossible for us in Scotland to get artificial limbs unless we employed alien limbmakers who were already at work in this country. Having unbounded confidence in the potentiality of Glasgow, and in the capacity, youth and vigour of her sons, I have no hesitancy in saying that even were we left without professional limbmakers we would still get, in such a cause, those who would make artificial limbs sufficient for the demand.

"Why, we have men here whose creative genius has made the Dreadnoughts possible and others who call into existence the lightest, fastest ships afloat, and whose works are as dreams realised of what physics may create for us. …We have …men who are used to work and fit to the 4000th part of an inch, to whom artificial limbs must appear but primitive conceptions."

Those limbs were largely made from willow and thereby hangs a much-loved tale of Macewen's habit of ignoring petty concerns which hindered the solving of a problem. Sir Donald MacAlister, principal of Glasgow University's account bears retelling. He met Macewen in the university grounds "standing before two old trees of no great sightliness."

Asked what he was thinking about, Macewen replied: "We are short of willows for artificial limbs at Erskine. Can I have these?" MacAlister's reply, that he was sure the university court would donate them if asked, was enough for the surgeon in a hurry. "If you are sure of that, I'll ask afterwards," he said. The trees disappeared that afternoon and Sir Donald could not recall any request ever coming before the court.

The Vanishing Willows, the title of John Calder's 1982 history of Erskine perfectly captures not only Macewen's practical approach but the spirit with which he imbued Erskine. Happily, the evocative phrase lives on in the name of the tearoom attached to the commercially-run garden centre at the gate of the Erskine estate.

Many regarded Macewen as autocratic; he was evidently impatient with what he saw as unnecessary obstacles and his success and prestige made him confident of his own abilities. First World War veterans at Erskine have spoken of his ebullient bedside manner. "He used to tell us that Macewen and God, in that order, would see us right." It is difficult to gauge the nuances of this in a completely different society but it seems likely it was intended as a combined morale booster and warning that there were no guarantees.

The sheer number of amputees who lived productive and relatively independent lives is testament that he did, indeed, "see them right."

Macewen was elected president of the British Medical Association "with acclamation" in 1922 and remained Regius Professor of Surgery at the University of Glasgow until his death, in Garrochty, Isle of Bute, on March 22, 1924. In the obituary carried in The Glasgow Herald, Dr Freeland Fergus described him as "a born investigator, one very little controlled by received opinion or by authority, no matter how great, for he was a man who instinctively looked at things from a critical point of view and brought all his extraordinary powers of keen observation to bear on every subject he touched."

As his biographer AK Bowman noted in 1942 (The Life and Teaching of Sir William Macewen – a chapter in the history of surgery), although originally simply a member of the civic committee to establish the hospital, "Macewen became the presiding genius and spirit of the place. The rise of Erskine Hospital, the evolution of its special work and all that it stands for today, was the fruit of his vision, practical foresight and organising and technical ability." The extent of his remarkable foresight becomes even more apparent with the realisation that these words, written half way through the Second World War, hold true 100 years on as Erskine provides continuing care and rehabilitation for veterans of armed conflict, even into old age.

Princess Louise, its first royal patron, unable to be present to unveil the memorial to Macewen at Erskine in 1925, wrote "The Hospital was Sir William's special child, which he created and put his whole heart and soul into." The hospital he created has been replaced by homes providing comfortable, 21st century facilities for disabled and elderly service veterans but the sympathetic care and encouragement he prescribed remain central. There could be no more fitting memorial to a unique man, showered with honours for advances in medical science but remembered fondly by his patients for his compassion.

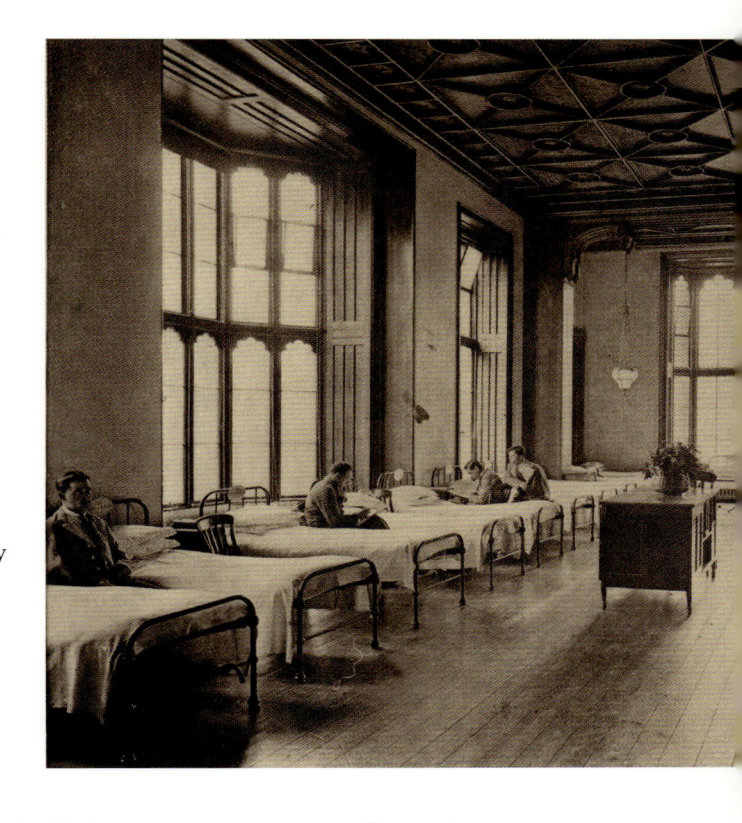

The grand rooms were transformed into wards with rows of hospital beds for amputees.

Sir Harold Yarrow

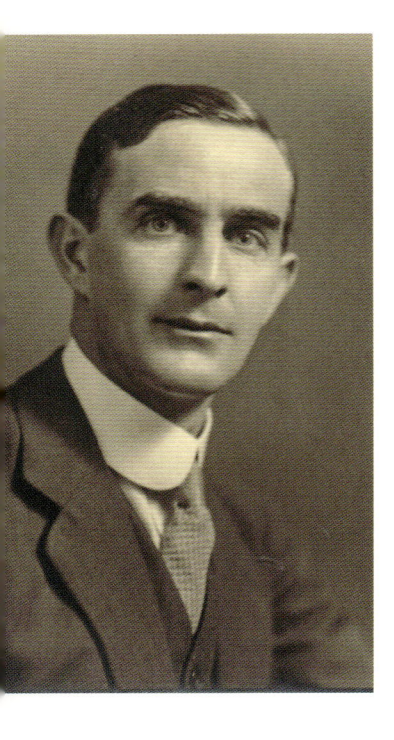

In 1919, eight of Erskine's double amputees demonstrated walking, running and dancing before an astonished audience at the Key Industries Exhibition. Three climbed ladders for an encore.

A portrait of Sir Harold from the 1920s.

The 1924 Minutes of the Limbs and Appliances Sub-Committee noted that from a total of 7,795 patents treated at Erskine since October 1916, 6,392 had been fitted with artificial limbs and ventured: "This is a noteworthy record for an industry that had to be created in haste."

That is surely an understatement. At the meeting convened by Sir William Macewen in Glasgow's City Chambers on March 29 1916, to propose the creation of a Scottish hospital to cater for military amputees, he scorned the idea that Scotland was incapable of creating from scratch an industry to serve the thousands of maimed Scottish soldiers returning from the trenches: "Why, we have men here whose creative genius has made the Dreadnoughts possible and others who call into existence the lightest, fastest ships afloat…. We have real men all around us accustomed to do things; who have clear brains used to invent all sorts of appliances and skilled hands capable of carrying their ideas into fruition."

Sir William knew well that there was one man in his audience who was already primed to answer his call. Harold Yarrow, at age 30, had taken over management of his father, Sir Alfred Yarrow's yard at Scotstoun in 1914. The yard was ideally placed to begin mass production of warships. (By 1918 it had turned out 29 of the fastest destroyers in the world, as well as a gunboat, a submarine and three hospital ships, all for the Royal Navy.)

Harold had already been warned by his father that Britain faced an unprecedented crisis regarding the production of artificial limbs. Yarrow Senior had visited Chelsea Hospital several times, where amputees were being fitted with limbs being made by an American team based at Roehampton. Sir Alfred was unimpressed by the scale and quality of the operation and ordered 50 sets of artificial limbs from Japan, which had specialised in prosthetics, in response to the need created by its war with Russia. And Harold was looking at limbs used by the London and North-West Railway Co., which had enabled men injured in line-side accidents to return to work.

Meanwhile men who had required amputations were pouring in from the Western Front and elsewhere and faced long waits for artificial limbs, delays that were damaging both physically and psychologically. The use of ligatures and antiseptic might mean that men, who would have died of their wound a century before, now survived. However, the deadly accuracy and destructive power of a new generation of armaments were producing casualties on an unprecedented scale. And the mud of the Western Front, combined with the concentration of men and animals cheek by jowl in primitive living quarters, provided the perfect breeding grounds for infections, infections that could turn a survivable wound into a fatal one and which resulted in many thousands of amputations that could have been avoided in other conditions.

When Sir William took up the cudgels on behalf of Scottish amputees, he knew that Scotland's industrialists and landed gentry would back him. Why? Their own sons and brothers were among the victims of this ghastly war and they were looking for ways to "do their bit."

Harold Yarrow had been one of the select few invited to an initial meeting, held at the Faculty Hall of the College of Surgeons in Glasgow in early autumn 1915 to float the idea of a Scottish hospital to treat and care for amputees. So was Professor Archibald Barr, the brilliant engineer, who had given up his chair at Glasgow University to concentrate on building the world-renowned company of Barr and Stroud, based in Anniesland. When Harold agreed to chair the Limbs and Appliances Sub-Committee, he invited to join him not only his own wife Eleanor, who came from a family of well-known philanthropists, but also Archie Barr and his wife Isabella.

Before the war the Barrs at Westerton of Mugdock and the Yarrows of Campsie Dene House in Blanefield, were both involved in the setting up of Strathblane Village Club, the community venue that thrives to this day. But by March 1916, when we have the rather dry first minutes of the Limbs and Appliances Sub-Committee, the Barrs and the Yarrows were bound together by far more than the usual professional and social links.

Sir Alfred had wanted his youngest son, Eric, to join Harold in running the Scotstoun yard. Eric had pleaded with his father to allow him to join up, arguing: "There are many of the working class who are sacrificing a great deal by enlisting." By early 1915, Eric had joined the Barr's brilliant son Jack, a recent Oxford graduate, in Northern France where both had been commissioned into the 7th Argyll and Sutherland Highlanders as second lieutenants. Letters and photographs show two young men making the best of things and enjoying their time off together until April 25 when Jack was killed during an attack near Ypres. After dark, Eric Yarrow crawled into no-man's land, found his best friend and carried the body to a grave he had dug behind the lines. His long heartfelt letters of condolence to the Barr family culminate on May 7 in one to Jack's sister Morag in which he contrasts the shattered landscape around Ypres with the beauty of the Blane valley where "although the walls of our fair homes stand intact, the hearts of the inhabitants are broken." Eric Yarrow was killed in a surprise attack the following day.

It is against this emotional backdrop that one should read the prosaic minutes of the Limbs and Appliances Sub-Committee. In April, Harold reports that arrangements were being made for the supply of willow, a wood that combined strength and lightness, and the creation of limbs was to be centralised at the pattern shop in Yarrows, with some orders sub-contracted to other Clydeside firms. Joiners at Yarrows' pattern shop had managed to produce the first prototypes within 48 hours, using the limbs supplied by the railway company. These were passed as acceptable by the Medical Board of the War Office.

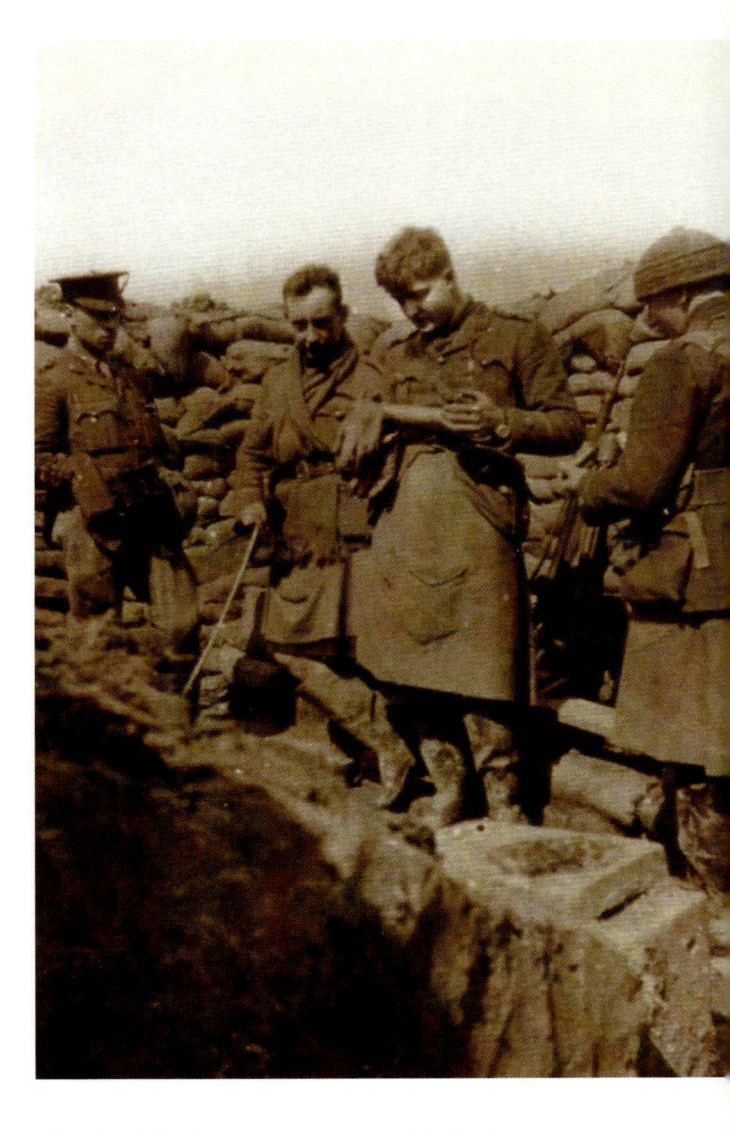

Snapshot of Jack Barr and Eric Yarrow together in an Argyll Trench near Messines shortly before their deaths in April/May 1915.

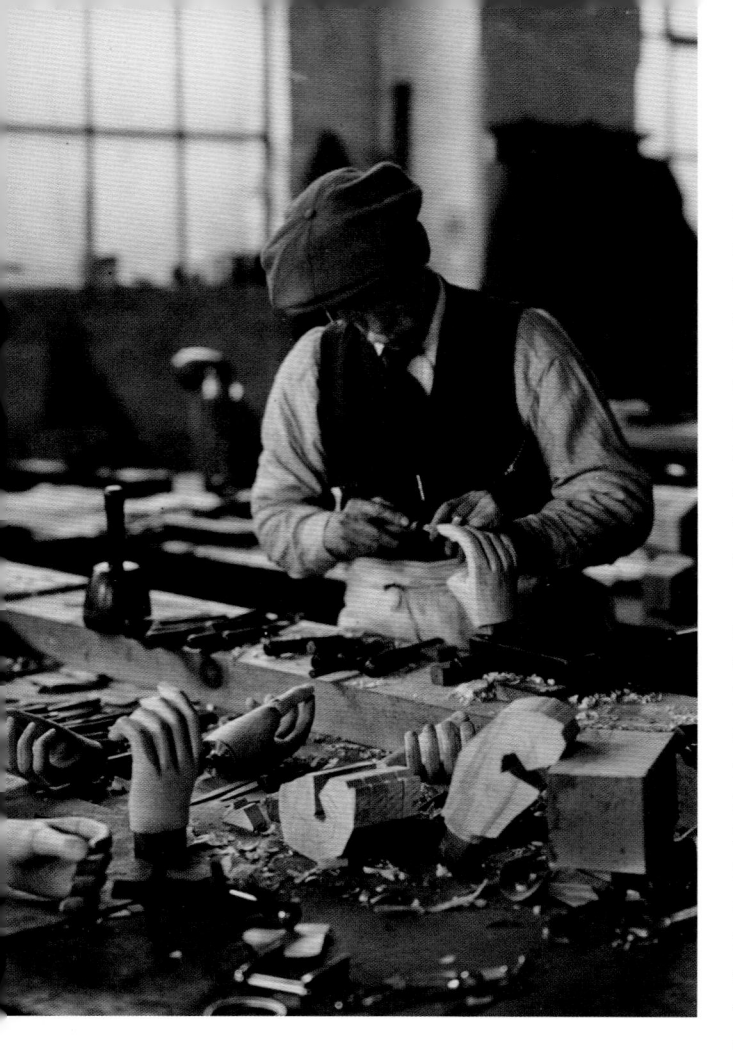

A man carving an artificial hand in the Pattern fitters shop at Yarrow Shipbuilders.

As Harold Yarrow would explain in a subsequent article (The Engineer, September 1918) an artificial arm presented an entirely different technical challenge to that of an artificial leg. The dilemma for the arm was that it needed to look sufficiently like the real thing so as not to attract attention when protruding from the sleeve of a shirt or jacket. At the same time, it needed to be functional and at that time, there was little to beat a well-made hook. The solution for early Erskine patients (see the chapter on Corporal James Ritson) was to supply both, each with a screw or bayonet joint attached to the leather bucket on the stump into which the artificial hand or the hook could be affixed to meet the circumstances.

Legs were more complicated, mainly because they often needed to accommodate knee as well as ankle joints and they needed to be weight-bearing. They also needed to be light, durable and comfortable. A well-made, well-fitted, comfortable limb literally put a man on his feet again, ready to take up his place again in the home and in the workplace. It meant that in his own mind he was no longer "a cripple." For above the knee amputation, the limb consisted of a bucket fashioned to fit the stump, strong elastic to mimic the action of the knee and a willow foreleg and foot jointed at the ankle with sturdy springs. The knee joint used a strong steel bolt and leather bushes. The weight of the seasoned wood is less than half its previous weight and far lighter than the human limb.

Soon a third of the pattern shop at Yarrows was given over to the design and manufacture of arms and legs. But how to find enough seasoned willow to go into full production? Usually seasoning alone took a year. Again, necessity proved the mother of invention. The Yarrow patternmakers discovered that by boring holes through two-foot sections of willow and carefully drying them over electric fans to prevent cracking, fully seasoned wood could be secured in two to three weeks.

Where could so much willow (or 'saugh' in Scots) be sourced so quickly amidst the prevailing wood shortage? Easy. Yarrow and Macewen's appeal to the great and the good produced cartloads of the stuff. The minutes record: "Lord Blythswood has donated 25 willows; Sir George Stirling of Glorat has offered large numbers of willow from his estate; 14 willows from Marquis of Ailsa, Culzean" et cetera.

By November 1916, such was the demand for prosthetic limbs that Harold Yarrow had gathered what would be known as the Clyde Consortium of Limbs Makers. They included Ailsa Shipbuilding Co Ltd in Troon (where Erskine's first patient had worked as a rigger), the Fairfield Shipbuilding Co Ltd, Wm Denny and Brothers, William Beardmore and Co Ltd, the North British Loco Ltd, and WB Hilliard and Sons. By the following June the Ayrshire Dockyard Co of Irvine, John Brown & Co Clydebank, Scotts of Greenock and Linthouse in Govan had all joined. And none of these companies ever turned a penny profit from the venture. All work was carried out on a cost only basis: "the chief desire being to render some assistance to the limbless men who have fought for their country." (The Engineer, Sept 1918)

Asked to put a cost on producing each limb, Yarrow and his committee settled on £11 per leg (later raised to £12) regardless of whether amputation was above or below the knee and agreed the fee with the Chelsea Commissioners. The charge for a forearm was £7.

Within five months of opening its door Erskine Hospital had provided 94 men with artificial limbs, each personally fitted on site in the hospital workshop.

With typical foresight Yarrow worked hard to produce standardised steel parts, which would become important for repair and maintenance. Feedback from the Ministry of Pensions was encouraging.

In December 1917 the committee agreed to provide artificial limbs to three female munitions workers Ena Walker, May McIvor and Rose Ann Wilson, injured in workplace accidents.

In March 1918 the Prince of Wales visited Yarrows and was shown the limb-making taking place in the pattern shop. The Glasgow Herald reported: "Mr Yarrow explained the process of manufacture to the prince, who closely examined one of the limbs."

By 1919 the hospital had started accumulating thank-you letters from men who had been using the limbs for two years. Providing each patient with an Erskine Provisional Limb on admission did away with the need for crutches, enabling men to move on to a permanent limb more quickly. In the same year eight of Erskine's double amputees demonstrated walking, running and dancing before an astonished audience at the Key Industries Exhibition. Three climbed ladders for an encore.

By 1920 the "Erskine Limb" was winning plaudits for its lightness and durability. By then only six of the Clyde Consortium put together by Harold Yarrow were still making limbs but the flow of patients continued. Some of these men would require "re-amputations" after the crude butchery of a field hospital under pressure, or the removal of necrotised bone or shrapnel from limbs or torso.

In 1924, by which time all limb production and repair was being done in the Erskine workshop, the committee reported that from a total of 7,795 patents treated at Erskine since October 1916, 6,392 had been fitted with artificial limbs and ventured: "This is a noteworthy record for an industry that had to be created in haste."

For some patients there would be many return visits to Erskine, while others trotted off on their Erskine Limb with barely a backwards glance. The article in the Engineer Magazine recorded a man who had recently re-visited the hospital. Despite having had both of his legs amputated below the knee, he was now continuing his old profession as a window cleaner.

The 1920s were difficult times for Yarrows as the inevitable post-war collapse in warship orders forced a re-focus on boiler-making with a much scaled down workforce. But Harold Yarrow still found time for Erskine where times were equally hard. In 1926 when he became Honorary Treasurer and Convenor of the Finance Committee, the accounts were already in the red. Veterans needed to return to the hospital for adjustments to their artificial limbs. There were 150 admissions that year and Erskine was also the permanent home of a number of severely disabled men, who found employment in the various workshops (including men

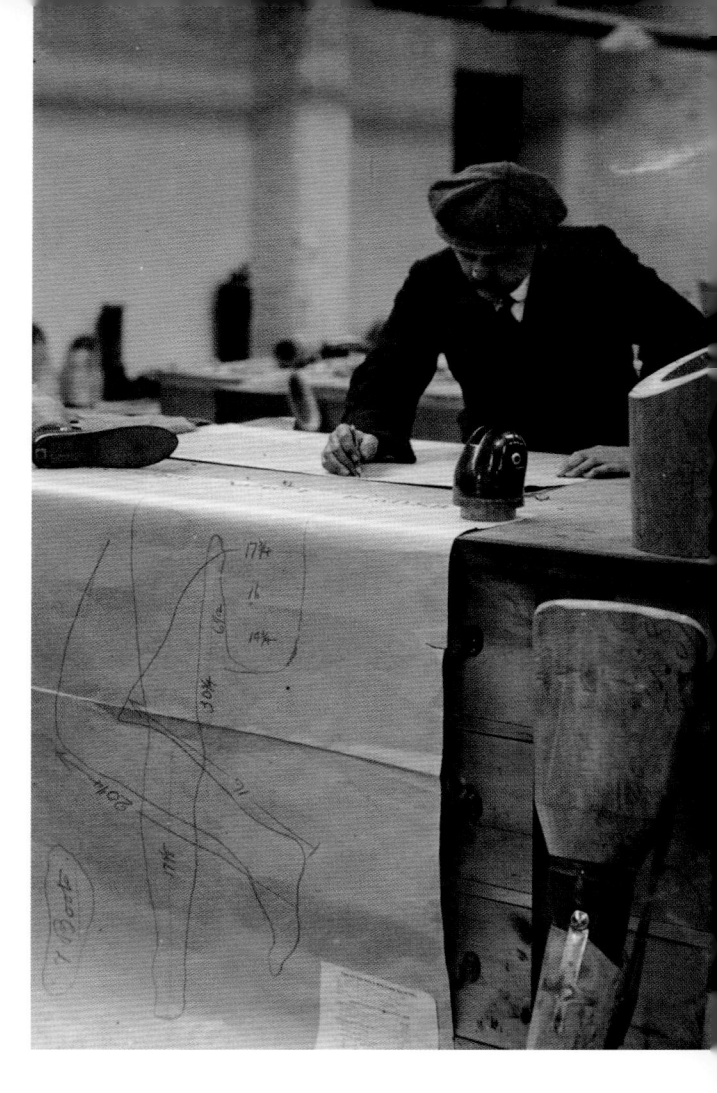

The limb fitters' wokshop at the hospital.

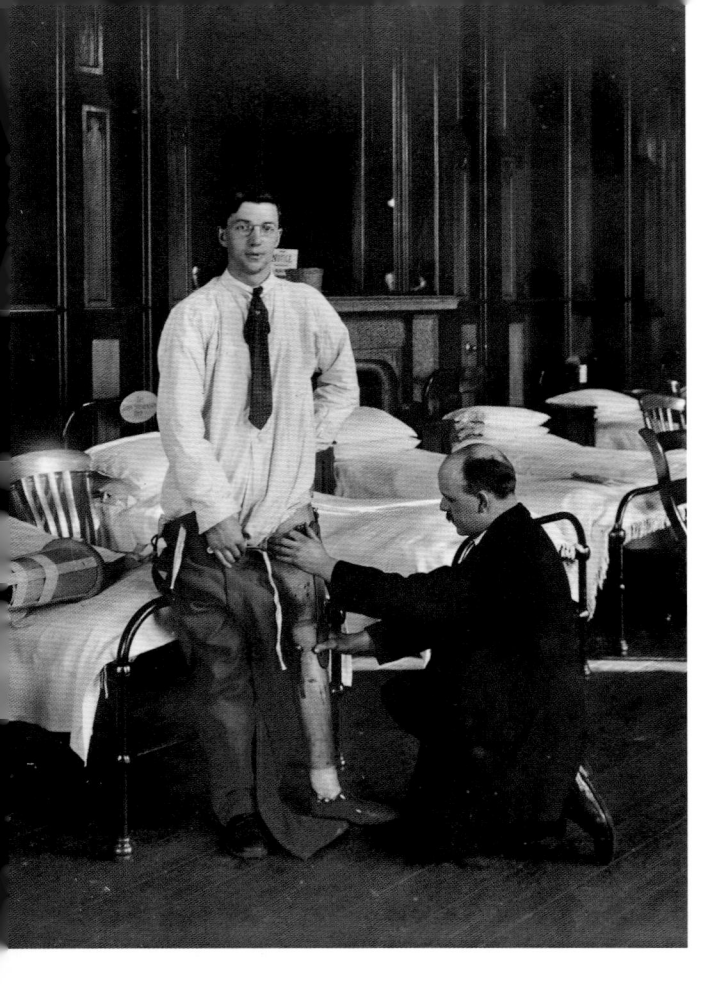

An artificial limb being adjusted by a limb fitter.

without arms or with advanced stage heart disease, who were deemed "100% disabled"). The workshops never turned a profit. That wasn't the point. And while some on the executive regarded these workshops as an unaffordable drain on resources, Harold Yarrow staunchly defended them: "The value of the actual output of goods must bring home to all the sense of brave effort, amazing pluck and steady endurance on the part of the heavily-disabled ex-servicemen and a wonderful strength of resolution to carry on."

But as the First World War receded in the memory and global recession began to bite, there was a risk that the Scottish public would wear their poppies on Remembrance Day but forget disabled war veterans for the rest of the year. In the hope of tackling the deficit, Yarrow took to the airwaves on Christmas Day 1927 with a broadcast appeal, then something of a novelty.

In 1940, with Germans bombs falling in and around Erskine and despite the workload of a shipyard in full production, Yarrow, now Sir Harold, following the death of his father eight years earlier, took on the daunting task of chairing the hospital's Executive Committee. The Princess Louise Hospital, as Erskine was then known, was now taking in freshly wounded personnel, as well as caring for severely disabled permanent residents and old soldiers from the First World War in need of support in their final years. Again Yarrow launched a public appeal and again the Scottish public rallied around. Nearly £54,000 was raised, two-thirds of it raised by sales to a parched nation of whisky donated by various branches of the spirits trade.

Yarrow was still chairman in 1947 when the advent of the National Health Service presented an existential dilemma to Erskine. Would it be nationalised and become part of the new service or retain its cherished independence?

Sir Harold and his committee battled behind the scenes and they won. In March 1948 a letter was received informing them that the Secretary of State for Scotland had decided that "the transfer of the hospital will not be required for the purposes of providing hospital and specialist services."

Meanwhile Sir Harold was also chairing a sub-committee considering the post-war requirements of the hospital, including new operating theatres, occupational therapy facilities, a convalescent wing and a hostel for workshop employees.

Even in the mid-1950s and now in his 70s, he was still Honorary Treasurer and a member of the Executive Committee but by now another generation was preparing to offer its services to Erskine. Harold and Eleanor's only son, born in 1920, was named Eric for his uncle who had died on the Western Front five years before.

History would repeat itself in 1939, when young Eric could have opted to join the Yarrows payroll or continue with his studies but felt uncomfortable in Civvy Street, when all his pals were joining up. So he joined the Royal Engineers and, as a major, went on to a distinguished military career in the Far East. (This included blowing up in the Irrawaddy delta several ships made at Yarrows.)

"My father always told me he hoped that Erskine was one of the charities I would support when he was no longer there," said Sir Eric Yarrow, who celebrated his 95th birthday in 2015. He barely needed to be asked: "I think I was on the executive when he was still alive." (Sir Harold died in 1962.)

As well as leading the company founded by his grandfather and which had produced 1,283 ships in 112 years, prior to the yard's nationalisation in 1977, Sir Eric took on the chairmanship of Erskine's Executive Committee in 1980. "I took over from General Gordon Macmillan. I said I had an awful lot on my plate but he said there was nothing in it. That was nonsense of course."

For the next six years, Sir Eric, who latterly also chaired the Clydesdale Bank, was a frequent visitor to Erskine, dashing off for meetings after a long day at the helm at Scotstoun, where he continued post-nationalisation. The opening of the Erskine Bridge in 1971 had been a blessing. "Before that it was a question of getting pally with the Erskine ferry people. They always managed to squeeze my car in."

Sir Eric tried to make executive meetings less formal and more businesslike. "Money was a constant source of worry, as it had been in my father's day. And like him, I very much encouraged the idea of the workshops." So in the 1980s, the son was making the same argument his father had made half a century before: that they provided essential employment and motivation for Erskine's long-stay residents, even though by this time each worker cost the charity more than £3,000 a year.

Annual reports from his time as chairman reveal a constant struggle to balance the books, as capital reserves were eroded by inflation.

A generous Scottish public continued to keep Erskine afloat. In 1984, for example, though 33% of income came from board charges, 5% from investment income and 18% from government departments, 44% came from legacies and donations.

And there was another looming problem. As Sir Eric put it in his first annual report: "We have the problem of providing a Hospital, which can fulfil all the clinical and therapeutic requirements and which can also serve as a Home." This was a conflict that was never resolved until the re-birth of Erskine essentially as a care home, with state of the art facilities and individual rooms, in addition to cottages in the grounds for disabled ex-service personnel and their families.

During his chairmanship Sir Eric married his third wife, Joan, who duly joined the General Council at Erskine and has continued the Yarrow connection, which now goes back 100 years. Lady Yarrow's tasks have ranged from pushing around the library trolley to helping decide what to salvage when Erskine made the big move from the mansion house into brand new facilities in 2000. Sir Eric has spent two spells of respite care at Erskine after falls and remains a great fan: "They are excellent at keeping people occupied. I played bingo and gave a talk about Burma. When I go, it'll be Donations to Erskine, if desired."

Today prosthetics have moved into a new era. One wonders what Corporal James Ritson with his Clyde-built forearm, would have made of a bionic arm produced using 3-D printing technology and which relays movement to a robotic hand from sensors picked up from an electronic signal produced by flexing the arm muscles. Today men are able to run on their prostheses, in some cases faster than a competitor on two legs. Casualties from recent conflicts in Iraq and Afghanistan are once more pushing prosthetic technology forward.

But we should never forget the gentleman's agreement between a pioneering surgeon and an enterprising businessman, mourning the death of his young brother, that put thousands of maimed Scottish soldiers and sailors back on their feet again – feet made of willow, the wood that put the "sauch" into Sauchiehall Street.

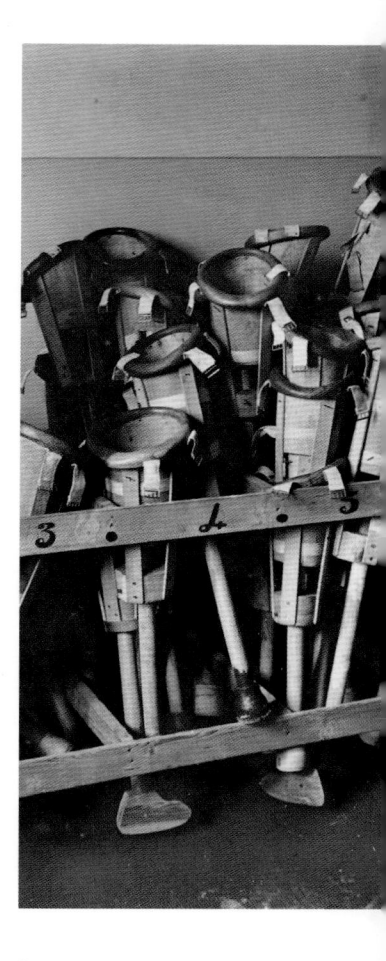

Provisional limbs arranged in different sizes so as to be readily accessible.

James Ritson

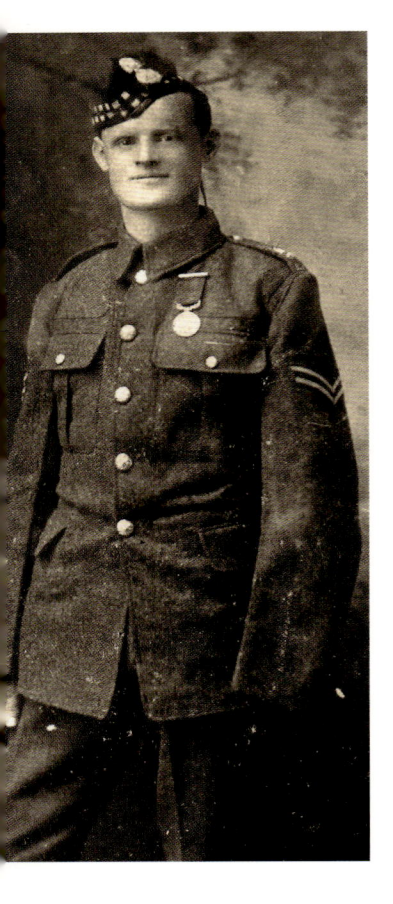

"A great number of my comrades fell at Gallipoli and will never return, so that it may be said that I have been fortunate in emerging from such an ordeal with only the loss of my left hand."

Who was Erskine's very first patient? According to the admissions book for what was then unsparingly described as "The Princess Louise Scottish Hospital for Maimed and Limbless Sailors and Soldiers", it was Corporal J Ritson of the 1/5th Royal Scots Fusiliers, a 29-year-old rigger from Troon in Ayrshire.

In fact, 14 patients were admitted to the hospital on that day, October 10, 1916 but Jimmy Ritson has the honour being first in the huge admissions book, a tome that would last into the 1930s. And, as it happens, his life is a story well worth the telling.

He was born in Barrow-in-Furness in Cumbria on February 28, 1887, the son of a platelayer. He appears to have joined the Royal Navy at around age 15 and served for eight years, winning prizes for boxing. So by the time he stepped ashore in Troon in 1909, he already boasted a powerful physique. As his son David puts it: "He jumped on a boat, landed in Troon and fancied my mother."

Helen Shannon had had a hard life. She was born in Anderston Glasgow in 1886 to a Scots-Irish couple, Samuel Shannon, described as an iron ship plater, and his wife Margaret. Helen married William Dugan McCormick, a 21-year-old labourer in Troon in 1907. They had two children, James and Margaret, before William sailed off to Canada to seek work and seemingly died within a fortnight of disembarking, leaving Helen a widow at 23.

The 1911 Census describes her as a 25-year old widow, letting out rooms in her home at 1 Harbour Road, Troon. It looks likely that Jimmy Ritson found lodgings with her and they had a whirlwind affair. The couple were married in November 1911 and their first child, Mary Jane, arrived four months later. Jimmy took work in the Ailsa Shipbuilding Company Ltd in Troon, beginning as a plater's helper and latterly a rigger. He gained a reputation as a good and steady workman.

In 1914 at the outbreak of war, it would have been natural for Ritson to return to the RN but instead he volunteered for his local territorial regiment, the Royal Scots Fusiliers. David Ritson (his only surviving offspring in 2015) believes his father was awaiting his call-up from the Navy, when he was taunted in the street by three women, distributing white feathers to those perceived to be shirkers. If so, they must have been quick off the mark as Jimmy enlisted four days after Britain's declaration of war.

Initially he was stationed in Ayr, so able to make regular trips home. A breezy postcard to his sister signs off: "Tell them all I was asking for them. That's all at present as the cook house has sounded."

In October 1914, Jimmy was able to get back to Troon for the birth of his son Thomas (although the child apparently did not survive into adulthood). Though he describes himself

Portrait of Ritson minus his left fore-arm, proudly wearing his Distinguished Conduct Medal.

in the birth record as a private, a group photograph with the rest of D Company 1/5th RSF soon afterwards shows him sporting the stripes of a corporal.

By the time Jimmy and his battalion left Liverpool for Gallipoli in May 1915, Helen was expecting their third child, Sarah Jane, always known as Sadie.

As First Lord of the Admiralty, Winston Churchill had been calling for the opening up of an Eastern Front, by attacking Germany's ally, Turkey, with the aim of ensuring a clear run into the Mediterranean through the Dardanelles for the Russian fleet. Jimmy and the RSF landed in Gallipoli on June 7 and were soon in the thick of the action. From the start it was obvious that the Turks were better armed and organised than anticipated and were determined to defend their home turf.

Matters came to a head on July 12 when the 4th and 5th RSF, along with the 4th and 5th King's Own Scottish Borderers were involved in an attack on a front between Kereves Dere and Achi Baba Nullah, near Krithia and sustained heavy losses.

Initially the 5th RSF were held in reserve but the main attack resulted in so many casualties that the remnants were too weak to attack the enemy fire trench and Jimmy and his comrades were sent in to consolidate ground already taken. Later it would be reported that when the officer in charge was wounded, Ritson "stepped forward and took command of the bombers, leading them in many desperate attacks." And when on July 13 an officer of the 7th Highland Light Infantry fell in front of the trenches, "Corporal Ritson rushed out and picked him up and carried him back over three of the trenches which they had taken from the enemy and brought him into safety." This gallantry would earn him the Distinguished Conduct Medal, second in importance only to the Victoria Cross.

On December 19 he was mentioned in dispatches for leading a bombing party that took a communications trench without the loss of a single man. Ten days later he was in action again, taking 20 prisoners and leading an attack on an enemy trench. This action would earn Jimmy Ritson a second DCM, in the form of a Bar.

However, the following day a Turkish mine exploded in Ritson's bombing pit. Everyone was injured or killed and Ritson was buried alive for some time. It was reported: "Corporal Ritson was buried in the debris and had to be dug out, when it was found that he had twenty-two wounds in his body. One of these proved to be so serious that he had to have his left hand amputated."

It is hard to believe that any human being could survive such injuries. Back home in Troon, Helen (now mother to five children under nine) received a brutally blunt pro forma letter from the Territorial Force Record Office, informing her that her husband had been evacuated by Hospital Ship HMS Gloucester to a military hospital in Malta, "suffering from multiple bomb wounds, both shoulders, left fore-arm blown off (Severe)." The comment in parenthesis seems rather superfluous.

Jimmy himself spoke little afterwards of how he survived what must have been months of torment, except to recall that immediately after the amputation, his stump was cauterized by being plunged into a bucket of hot tar. Like many other Gallipoli survivors, afterwards he had little time for Churchill and used to say: "Churchill was up above and we were down below like peas in a pod being blown to smithereens. The best thing the British did was get out of there and the Turks didn't even know it."

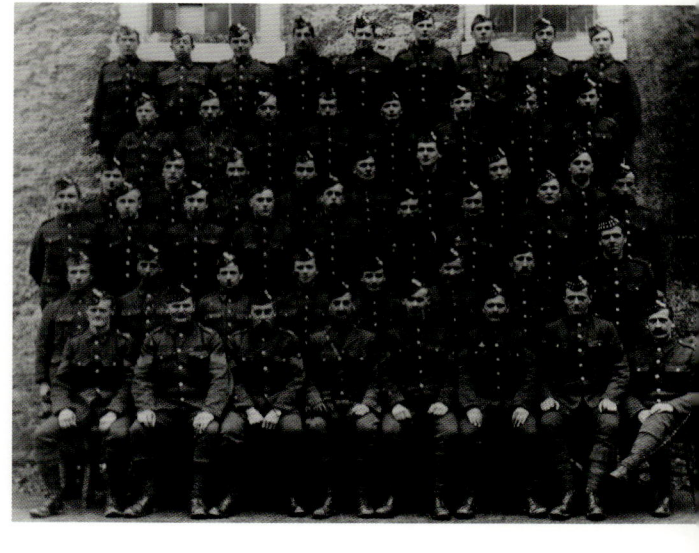

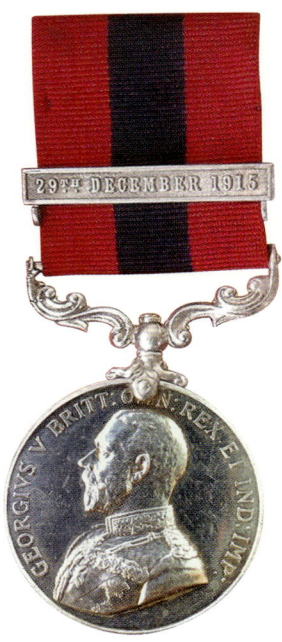

Top: Ritson with D Company Royal Scots Fusiliers 1/5th (front row, far left).

Above: Ritson's Distinguished Conduct Medal. His second honour is denoted by the Bar.

James Ritson 29

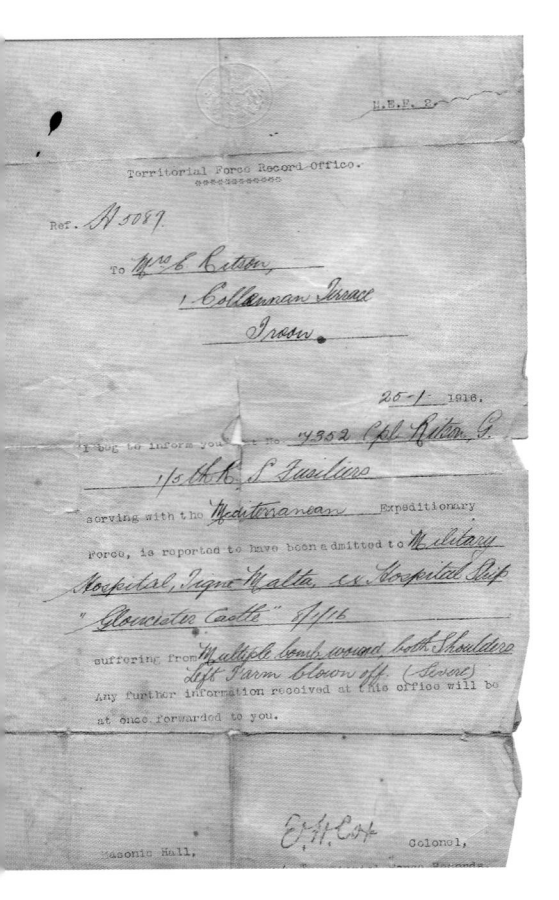

Ritson's honourable discharge.

Military historians are inclined to agree. The invasion was a disaster but, by keeping the withdrawal plans secret, many Allied lives were saved from what could have been a rout.

Soon Jimmy Ritson was back in Troon where he was the talk of the town. His comrades and officers also recognised his heroism. A letter from Captain Patrick Lavelle of the RSF, still held by the Ritson family, says: "I was greatly pleased to see Ritson got a clasp to his medal. He thoroughly deserved it and more. He was one of the finest fellows in our Battalion."

Another note from a Troon comrade still out in Egypt with the 1/5th RSF adds with a sarcastic note: "We all join in sending you and the wife our best compliments and may you be long spared to enjoy the pleasure of your future life. A VC should have been your just reward but you know Jimmie, you are only a Fusilier."

On September 1 1916, the Troon and Prestwick Times reported: "One of the largest crowds that has ever assembled in Troon, congregated at the bandstand on the esplanade on Tuesday evening" to witness Corporal Ritson receiving his DCM with Bar from the wife of the Provost, Mrs Muir. (Unfortunately the report names him as John Ritson.) His commendations for bravery were rehearsed at length, with "(cheers)" regularly punctuating the story. In addition to his medal, he received £61 in government bonds and money from the Town Council and £81 7s from a collection among his former workmates at Ailsa's shipyard and engine works. (The equivalent today of more than £8,500.)

Jimmy Ritson accepts these honours graciously: "A great number of my comrades fell at Gallipoli and will never return, so that it may be said that I have been fortunate in emerging from such an ordeal with only the loss of my left hand." (He is right. The 5th RSF lost around 160 officers and men in the attack near Krithia in mid-July 1915, with 140 more wounded.)

The Troon celebration finishes with Auld Lang Syne, a concert from the pipe band of the Royal Engineers and James Ritson being carried on the shoulders of his comrades around the enclosure. There were even three cheers for Mrs Ritson, who must have felt slightly bemused in her seat amongst the dignitaries. One hopes that the ladies of the White Feather Movement felt suitably chastened.

On October 10, Jimmy Ritson became Erskine's first official patient. Replacing an arm is a fundamentally different proposition to fitting an artificial leg. While the arm does not need to be weight-bearing, it should be aesthetically pleasing enough to look natural as it extends from the arm of a shirt or jacket. However, the wearer also needs to be able to achieve basic tasks if he is to regain a measure of independence. As his son David recalls, this involved a double solution for Jimmy: "They gave him a sort of cleek, which clicked into a fitting on the stump for doing manual tasks but he also had a hand with artificial fingers and a glove to go on it. I remember new gloves would arrive each year. Naebody liked the stump. Sometimes he could take off his hand and tease us with it. I didn't like it at all."

Just over a month after he entered the hospital, James Ritson was back with his family and getting on with life. In November he was "honourably discharged" from the army as "unfit for further military service" and provided with a reference which described him as "an honest, sober and willing soldier, who has always been found attentive to duty. Military character – very good."

However, like so many survivors of the horrors of the First World War, he had difficulty reintegrating into civilian life. He was no longer able to take up his work in the shipyard, though he was still immensely strong. "Even with the one arm, he could throw three men over his shoulder," says David. (By coincidence, Ailsa was one of the yards that joined the Clyde consortium that would take on the mass production of thousands of prosthetic limbs.)

Jimmy continued to be honoured for his war service. After the war he was awarded the beautiful gold and blue Troon Medal and Freedom of the Burgh in recognition of his gallantry.

He opened an ironmongery in Troon but in the thin years after the Great War, it failed to thrive. For some time he operated a smallholding in Loans, near Troon, raising pigs and chickens and selling produce from a stall. But that too failed to generate a decent income.

Meanwhile, the family grew and grew to the point where Jimmy and Helen had produced a total of eight children, on top of Helen's two children by her first marriage. Helen, named for her mother, was born in 1917, followed by Martha in 1920, Annie Shannon in 1922 and Emma in 1924. Finally, in 1926 there was, David, the son he must have craved. But there was tragedy too. In 1928 Mary Anne, the couple's eldest daughter, by now a 15-year old domestic servant working at the Portland Golf Clubhouse in Troon, caught her dress on fire while cleaning grease from a stove. There are various versions of this story but according to the report in the Troon and Prestwick Times, instead of submitting to having the flames smothered by a blanket, the panic-stricken girl ran outside "with the result that the breeze fanned the flames and she was at once enveloped from head to foot." Passers-by removed their coats in an attempt to quench the flames but Mary Anne was so badly burned that she never recovered and died in Kilmarnock Infirmary on January 31.

Jimmy Ritson, the model soldier, was not always the model citizen. His stated determination to renounce alcohol after his son was born in 1926 was seemingly honoured more in the breach and he was not always a considerate husband. Helen sometimes had to muddle through with very little money.

Though he admired his father's war record, David as the sole surviving son must have found it hard living up to his father's expectations, despite the compensation of six lovely sisters. Jimmy Ritson was a hard act to follow. Too young to serve in the Second World War, David had a successful career with the Prestwick-based aircraft manufacturer Scottish Aviation Limited and supported both the British Legion and the local TA, as well as Erskine. For a time Jimmy and Helen lived in the Templehill area of Troon and after his wife's death Jimmy moved to Barassie. To the end he retained his upright military bearing. As well as his eight children (and two stepchildren), Jimmy Ritson had 14 grandchildren by the time he died aged 83 from a coronary thrombosis in 1970.

Grandchildren include Ronnie, who rose through the ranks to become a pit manager, David who worked as a shipwright, Jean who became a medical secretary and Maureen, a hospital lab technician. And there were at least 20 great-grandchildren too.

The local press, which had devoted yards of coverage to Corporal Ritson's DCM and Bar in 1916, failed to mark his passing beyond the customary funeral notice.

So Erskine's first patient, and Troon's remarkable war hero, was seemingly forgotten by all but his nearest and dearest. Perhaps, it was the Gallipoli factor. Though the Allies were victorious in 1918, Gallipoli would go down in history as an expensive and disastrous attempt to distract the Germans' attention from the stalemate on the Western Front and many British, Commonwealth and Empire soldiers paid for it with their lives. That failure should not detract from the extraordinary courage of men like Jimmy Ritson, Erskine's Number One Patient.

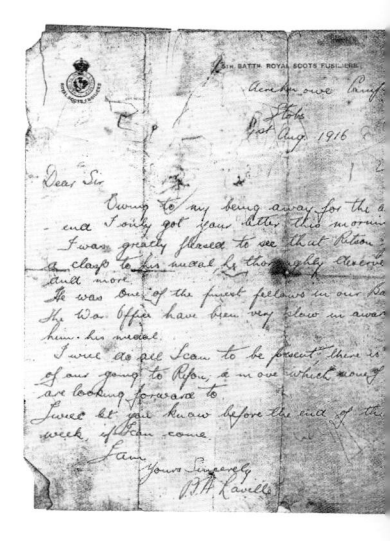

A letter from commanding officer Captain PJA Lavelle, expressing great pleasure upon hearing of Ritson's decorations.

Albert Young

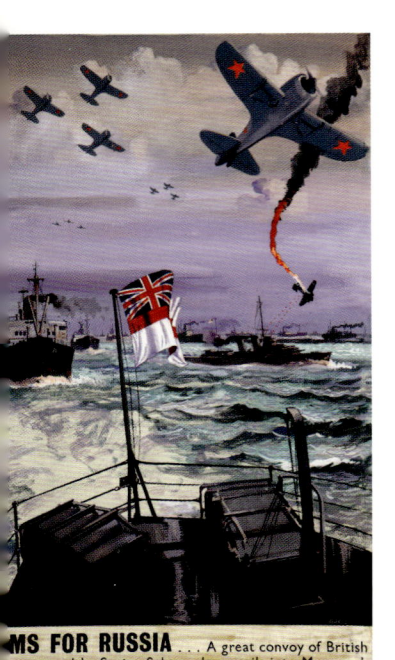

"Hitler had to be stopped. He wanted to rule the world and he got half way there too. We were only a small nation. We needed the Russians and they needed us."

British Government Arctic Convoys Poster from The National Archives.

There is a splendid oil painting on the wall of Albert Young's room at Erskine. It shows a destroyer called HMS Windsor ploughing through a choppy sea. The eye is drawn automatically to two tiny figures on the forward lookout station beside B gun. "That's me and my pal Guts," announces 96-year old Albert matter-of-factly. The painting is the work of his devoted nephew Ronald Young, who combines his artistic flair with a keen interest in World War Two naval history. The picture is a constant reminder of the story of Able Seaman Albert Edward Finch Young, a remarkable survivor.

It may be 70 years since the end of WW2 but interest in certain episodes in that conflict seems to grow each year. Recently there has been a renewed and horrified fascination with the Arctic Convoys in which thousands of British sailors ran the gauntlet of German bombers, warships and U-boats and some 3000 British seamen died in explosions, fires and ice cold seas in the interests of getting vital arms and supplies through to our Soviet allies. Winston Churchill once characterised the convoys as "the worst journey in the world", a harrowing passage in which ships risked capsizing on account of the weight of ice on their decks and rigging, when a grown man wept because his hands were too cold to work his gun, and when spending more than 20 minutes in Arctic seas was likely to be fatal.

The convoy that has lived longest in our collective memory was PQ17 in July 1942, when First Sea Lord Admiral Dudley Pond infamously ordered the armed escort to scatter, owing to the perceived threat from German surface ships. That left the Allied merchant ships to be picked off one by one by the Luftwaffe in the perpetual daylight of the Arctic summer. Only 11 out of 35 reached Russia and 153 merchant seamen lost their lives. Churchill later described PQ17 as "one of the most melancholy naval episodes in the whole of the war." Such was the scale of the disaster that the Admiralty temporarily suspended the convoys.

By the time Albert and his shipmates on board HMS Windsor were ordered to Loch Ewe to escort PQ18 in early September, news of the terrible fate of PQ17 had begun to circulate. "We knew lots of men had drowned but we didn't have time to be scared. We were under orders and just had to get on with it," says Albert.

Originally destined for the Russian port of Murmansk, at the last minute the Windsor was diverted to escort an offshoot of the main convoy, namely two oil tankers being sent across the Arctic Ocean to Spitzbergen for refueling purposes. "We set off two days ahead of the main convoy and got through scot-free." Though losses from PQ18 were smaller than its predecessor and the Allies regarded it as a success, 13 of the 41 ships involved were lost. An upbeat contemporary newspaper report headlined "ENEMY HARD HIT IN CONVOY", reported 40 aircraft and two U-boats had been destroyed during the operation despite the fact that "the enemy is in a position to attack from bases conveniently situated along the flank of the convoy route."

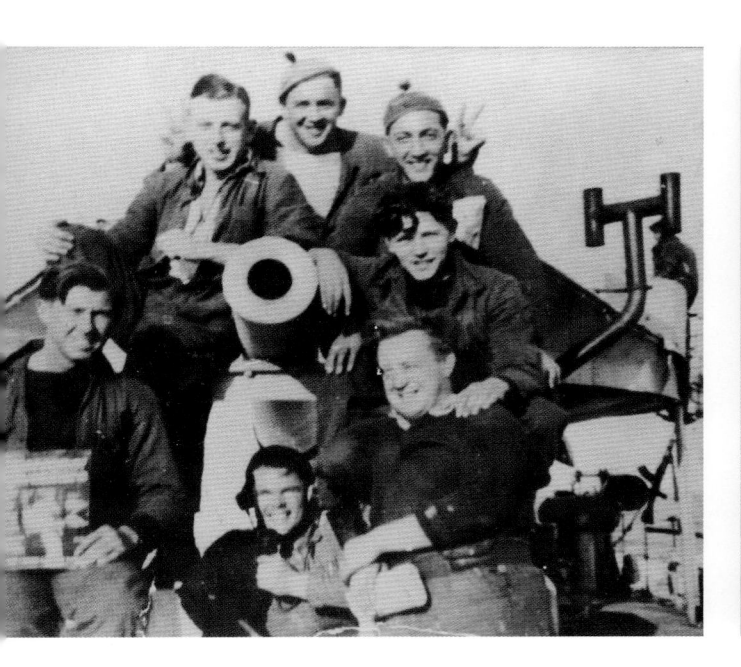

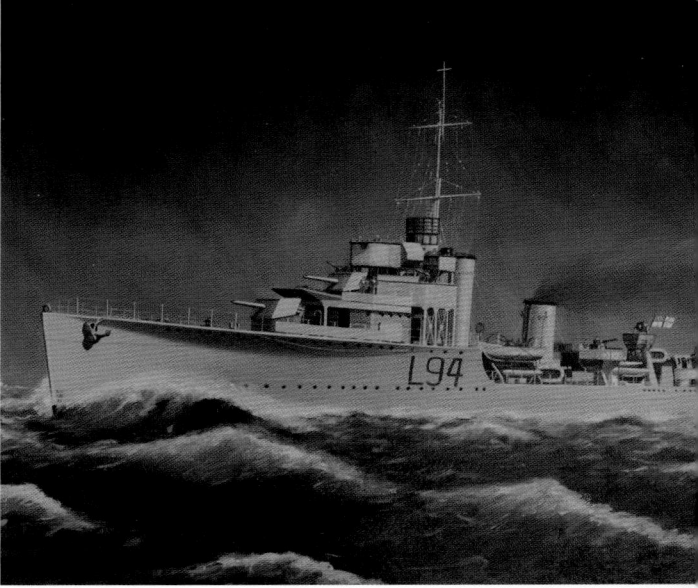

After accompanying the two oil tankers, the Windsor had been ordered to sail on and accompany the convoy returning from Archangel. "We were told to come up to HMS Somali, which had been torpedoed and was being towed by another Tribal class destroyer, HMS Ashanti. But a force ten storm blew up with waves higher than houses. The ships were pitching wildly with water constantly breaking over the decks. The force of it broke the Somali in two. She folded in half and sank. Most of the men in the water didn't stand a chance." Only 35 of the skeleton crew survived.

Wasn't it chilling to think that he could have been one of those drowning sailors? "No, I never thought that way," says Albert, who has always been fortified by his strong Christian faith rather than strong drink. (He confides: "I always took the threepence a day you could get instead of the rum ration.")

PQ18 was one a series of lucky escapes for Albert, whose war service sometimes reads like the portrait of a charmed life. (The superstitious might attribute this to him being the seventh son.) He was born on August 20 1919 in Bell Street, Renfrew where his father worked as a master joiner for local landowner Lord Blythswood. "Before I was born the family had lived in a lodge house on the Blythswood estate and my mother's job was to open the gates for trains coming by." Lord Blythswood sometimes called on the family and on one occasion memorably described Albert as "the beautiful baby."

As well as six older brothers, he had three sisters, which cannot have been easy when the family ended up in a three-roomed tenement flat. "It was OK because my oldest brothers were already away by then so there were only ever six children at home. There were two double bed recesses in the kitchen and a fold down bed. Mother and father had the bedroom to themselves."

Unsurprisingly young Albert enjoyed life outdoors: "I remember playing hopscotch and marbles outside the Robertson Park. I had a gird and cleek (hoop and stick). It ran down the hill one day into the (River) Cart. It must be there yet!"

There were summer holidays spent messing about in rowing boats in Tighnabruaich, which was reached by steamer from Renfrew in those days. Nine decades later Albert can still recognise and name the houses rented by the family and the nicknames they gave to certain streets, including "Toothache View" (which housed the local dentist).

Left: Albert (top left) with his mates during the war.

Above: Oil painting of the HMS Windsor featuring Albert and Guts, painted by his nephew Ronald Young.

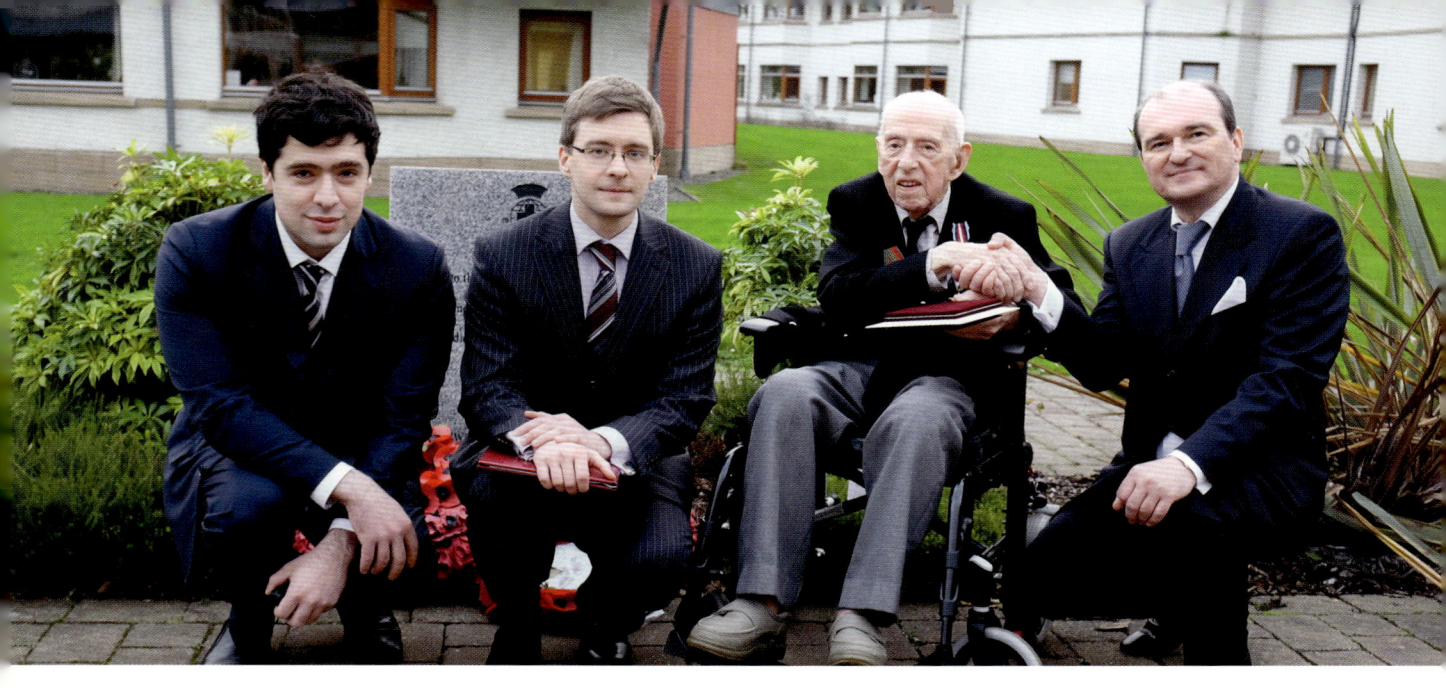

Andrew Pritsepov, the Consul General of the Russian Federation, with his two aides, presenting Albert with the Medal of Ushakov.

Albert's father was a well-known lay preacher at the Tent Hall in Glasgow. The young Albert was soon participating in church choirs and still enjoys singing hymns. At school he found he had a retentive memory. At 96 he retains an aptitude for spelling long words and can remember his Service Number: PSSX2070.

He left school at 14 and served an apprenticeship as a welder at Babcock & Wilcox but with two brothers in the merchant navy, he yearned for the sea. "I guess it was in my blood. At 17 ½ I signed up for the Royal Navy. I thought I'd get a strap on my back from my parents but they never said a word."

His first ship was HMS Tedworth, a Clyde-built coal-fired minesweeper, affectionately known as "Smokey Joe", which by coincidence had been launched at Renfrew two years before Albert's birth. But by the outbreak of WW2 he was serving on HMS Egret, a newly-built Royal Navy sloop, stationed in Aden. "War didn't frighten me one bit. We'd known it was imminent because in Port Said we fused all our live shells. Then we dropped off some Somali crew members on the way back to England. Later the Egret was sunk by a submarine. If I'd been on it then, I wouldn't be here talking to you."

But by then he was on HMS Windsor, a W-class destroyer built at Scotts of Greenock at the end of WW1. It would be his home for the next four years. As one of the older destroyers, it was used mainly for the vital role of convoy escorts, freeing newer vessels for combat.

Albert had two jobs. He was a quartermaster, which involved taking turns at the helm and piping people aboard. He was also captain of a Y gun (a reference to its basic shape). "When an attack was imminent they'd ring the bell on the mess deck like mad. It was the loudest bell I heard in my life. That was the signal for action stations. There were seven in our team and our job was to intercept German E-boats and try to stop them sinking Allied shipping. We sunk a German armed cruiser off the French coast once. When you fired on ships, you didn't want to see the seamen getting killed. It was the boat that you wanted to sink. It was a question of them or us."

Albert was helming the Windsor in May 1941 when some grim news came in: "HMS Hood had been sunk by the Bismarck, which was just out of the wrapper and the pride of the German fleet. We were ordered to escort the British battleship King George V and shield it from enemy fire. It helped sink the Bismarck a few days later."

Much time would be spent patrolling the North Sea, returning to Harwich at night to get

34 A Century Of Care: Erskine 1916 — 2016

orders for the following day. On one occasion the Windsor came under fire from a German armed cruiser and a shell hit the shield of Albert's Y-gun, setting it on fire. "I sent one of my gun crew to get a fire extinguisher and we managed to put it out. We had to be double quick because the blazing gun made us an obvious target." The man who put out the fire was Albert's pal John "Guts" Onslow (so-called because he was always hungry), who became a London fireman after the war.

Ironically, the Windsor sustained worse damage after being accidentally rammed by SS Methilhill, one of the ships in a convoy it was trying to protect. Come 1944 and the Windsor guarded convoys heading for the Normandy Beaches.

When did he start believing the Allies would win? "Pretty far on." In 1945 Albert ended up at HMS Armadillo, the commando base above Ardentinny on Loch Long.

Though he has seven medals, including three in connection with his role in the Arctic convoys, Albert would never mention it unless you did. "Five of us seven brothers were in the war. Hugh and Archie were in the merchant navy and Willie and Ian were in the army. I reckon my mother should have got the medals for letting the five of us go to war."

Albert was tempted to stay on in the RN. "They were offering £100, which was a lot of money then." But by now he had a good reason for staying ashore, in the shape of Martha, a girl he had met through his local church. They were married in Paisley in 1947.

Still itching for the sea, he took a job on a coal boat. "It was filthy. I lasted three days and then jumped ship at the Broomielaw in Glasgow without even waiting to get paid!" says Albert, who is rather fastidious. So he settled for his old welder's job and that was his career, working all over the UK and Northern Ireland. And he redirected his wanderlust into tramping the hills, continuing to walk up to 17 miles a day even at the age of 75. His fine bass voice graced the Rolls Royce male voice choir in East Kilbride. And he must be the oldest supporter of his local football team, Renfrew Juniors, who play barely a stone's throw from the site of his childhood home.

Though Albert and Martha (Mattie) did not have children, Albert is very close to his niece and nephew, Connie and Ronald and their respective families. Some years after Mattie's death, Albert took up residence at Orchard Court in Renfrew but moved to Erskine in 2014 when he began to need 24-hour care following diagnosis of Parkinson's disease. He settled in quickly and seems happy as the day is long. Each summer the family still take him on a nostalgia trip to Tighnabruaich and he enjoys simple pleasures, such as a weekly Auld's pie. "Or two. Even better!"

He takes pleasure in welcoming family and friends to his shipshape room at Erskine. In December 2014 he received an unexpected visit from a man he had never met: Andrey Pritsepov. The Consul General of the Russian Federation had come to present Albert with a coveted Ushakov Medal, in recognition of his role in the convoys. This followed a row between veterans' organisations and the UK Government, which had initially refused to allow those who had served in the convoys to receive a foreign honour. Albert politely abstained from this hullabaloo. It was not his style, even if he admits: "It was good of this chap to come all this way to pin a medal on me."

Though he doesn't see or hear too well these days, Albert is a great survivor. His old shipmates have all passed on. Guts Onslow died a few years back. And Albert's nine siblings have all gone too. As for HMS Windsor, she made her last journey, to the shipbreaker's yard in Charlestown, Fife in 1949.

How does Albert view the Arctic Convoys in an era when Germany feels more like an ally than Russia? "Hitler had to be stopped. He wanted to rule the world and he got half way there too. We were only a small nation. We needed the Russians and they needed us."

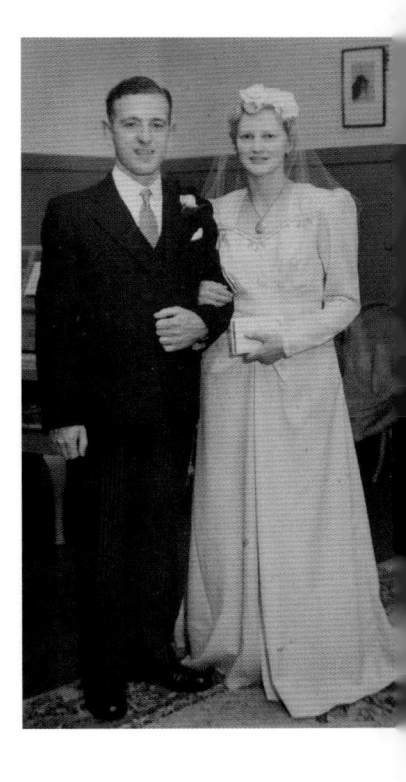

Albert and Martha on their wedding day in 1947.

Joe Parker

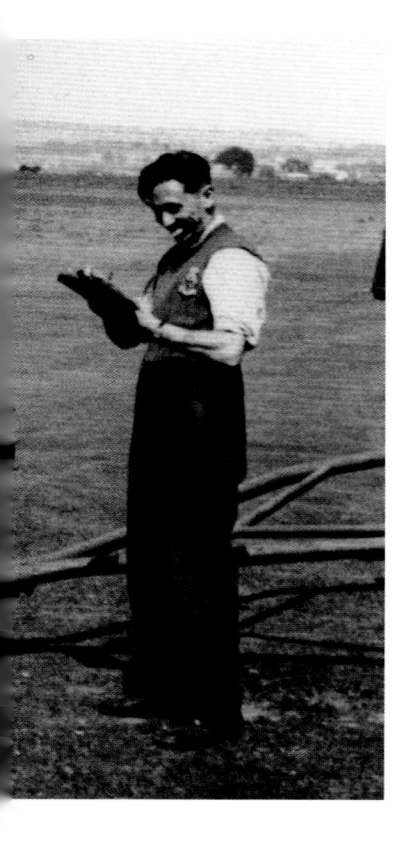

"The hood came down. Out jumped McKellar pumping his fists and shouting 'I got 'em!' Then we all piled into a car and rushed off to see the wreckage."

When a policeman turned up on the family's doorstep in Shettleston at 7am on August 23, 1939, Mr Parker feared his teenage son was in trouble. "What has he done?" he gruffly demanded, only to be mollified when the officer brandished Joe's Auxiliary Air Force call-up papers. To an 18-year old who was crazy about flying, it was like a dream come true. Instead of going off to work, he was going off to war.

"I was to report to Abbotsinch. The boys were all excited. It was a happy release for some of us. I had wanted to join the RAF at 16 but my parents wouldn't sign the papers. Instead I'd taken an apprenticeship as a toolmaker and then joined the City of Glasgow Auxiliary Air Force early in 1939. That meant spending two nights a week at the HQ in Glasgow across the road from the Plaza Ballroom and weekends at Abbotsinch, which wasn't much more than a group of wooden huts in those days." (A very far cry from its modern reincarnation as bustling Glasgow Airport.)

It was an exciting time for 602. In January it had been changed from an army co-operation squadron to a fighter unit and in May had taken delivery of a fleet of gleaming Spitfires, straight out of the packet.

"When the Prime minister announced on the wireless that Britain was at war with Germany, we all cheered. How naïve we were."

There followed a month of basic training, including "learning how to march properly" and then it was off to RAF Drem in East Lothian. "There were about 300 of us and six Spitfires ready to go at any one time. We were split into two groups working day on and day off. We went to bed in our clothes in a hut next to the planes. As soon as the alarm sounded, you were out on the runway getting the engines started up. Each plane had a seven-man team."

This meant Joe was witness to the first aerial action of the Second World War in British skies, when the Junkers of the Luftwaffe attacked British warships in the Firth of Forth on October 16 1939. Both 602 and 603 (City of Edinburgh) pilots brought down German bombers into the Forth estuary that day.

At this time Joe was aero engineer for Archie McKellar from Paisley, who would become Scotland's most celebrated Spitfire ace. The two men were already friends from their months together in the AAF. "He was a wee fella, like me (Joe is 5ft 3½ ins). He was very likeable. Always laughing and up to mischief. Some of the other pilots were a bit standoffish but Archie was like one of us. It wasn't unusual to be asked out for a drink."

On October 28 Joe waved Archie off on a second mission. Twelve days earlier McKellar had been involved in attacking one of the Junkers off Crail but the kill was given to another of 602's pilots, George Pinkerton. But this time the glory was all Archie's. Joe watched his pilot's return to base. He knew the guns had been fired because the red-painted flaps on the leading edge of its wings had turned black. "The hood came down. Out jumped McKellar

Joe at work on the airfield for 602 Squadron.

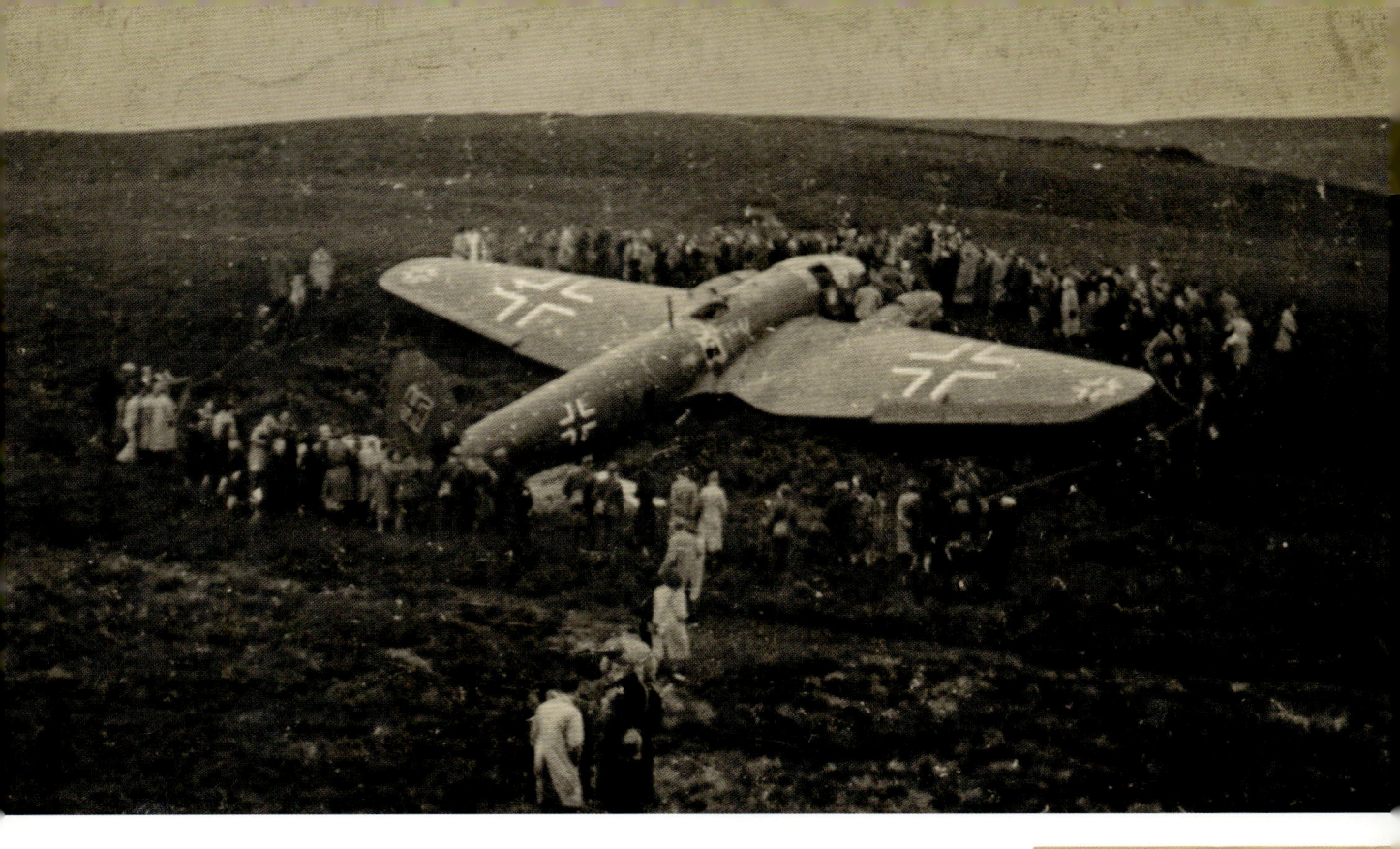

pumping his fists and shouting 'I got 'em!' Then we all piled into a car and rushed off to see the wreckage."

They found the pitted and holed, swastika-adorned Heinkel 111 lying askew on its crushed undercarriage near the village of Humbie in the Pentland Hills. "By the time we got there, there was quite a crowd of civilians. The crew came out with their hands up and I spoke with one of them: 'Why do you want to fight for Hitler?' I asked him. 'Why do you want to fight for Churchill?' he countered in perfect English. I couldn't believe it. He spoke with a distinctly Scottish accent. It seems his father had been something to do with the diplomatic service and he had spent part of his childhood in Scotland. I remember he called me 'Comrade'. And as the police took him away to be questioned, he said to me: 'For me the war is over. For you the war is just beginning.' After that it was more difficult to think of these men as the enemy. To be honest, they didn't seem very different from us."

Parts of the German plane are now on display at the 602 Squadron Museum in Glasgow. Joe too pocketed a piece of the aircraft as a souvenir.

By August 1940 602 Squadron was on the south coast of England preparing for the Battle of Britain "though of course, we didn't know it at the time. In Scotland it had been mostly like playing at being in the Air Force. But soon we were taking part in operations every day and there was night flying too. I was loving it."

Weren't there times when "his" Spitfire did not return? "Yes, there were. We felt gutted especially if we were friendly with the pilot but you just had to get over it. Usually you'd hear over the radio if your plane had been hit but 602 had a very high kill rate (89) and lost comparatively few of its own pilots. One day in a particularly tense dogfight 602 destroyed eight German fighters and shot down two others without losing a single pilot or aircraft.

"Quite often the pilot would turn up. I remember once down in Kent a pilot went missing. We heard he'd been shot down and everyone was feeling so sad. Then an ordinary bus drew up outside the base and out he came carrying his parachute. We were amazed.

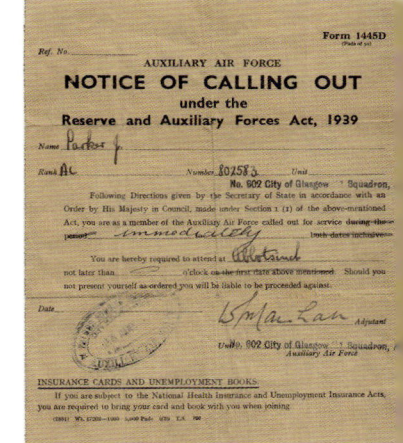

Top: The first German bomber brought down in Britain.

Above: Joe's call-out form.

Joe Parker 37

We had a party that night."

Joe's pal Archie McKellar was not so lucky. After chalking up 20 kills, he was killed in action on November 1 1940. To add insult to mortal injury, he was not listed on the Battle of Britain roll of honour in the RAF chapel at Westminster Abbey because he perished a few hours after the official end of the action.

As Joe speaks about this he lowers his voice and places one hand over his heart. "He had been promoted into another squadron by this time but I had a lot of feelings about his death because he had been one of the lads. No affectations."

Following the Battle of Britain Joe and 602 Squadron served at locations ranging from Orkney to Land's End. Whenever he could get away on a few days' leave, he would return to Glasgow to see his family. "The first Black American troops I ever saw were in Glasgow. They loved it here because they were treated as equals, while at home they had been separated."

Before the war, Joe had taken little interest in girls, preferring to take a bus into the country and tramp the hills around Glasgow with his pals on days off. "I felt inadequate. I thought I wasn't good enough, wasn't big enough, wasn't handsome enough to attract a girlfriend," he admits. But his smart uniform helped him grow, at least in confidence and on New Year's Eve 1940 he found himself standing opposite a petite and pretty girl called Jane Milroy at the Bobby Jones Ballroom in Ayr.

"I thought she'd not have time for me but I was wrong and we've got a daughter and two sons to prove it." Joe and Jane were married a few months later in Prestwick. The honeymoon was three days in a Glasgow hotel. "They were lots of hasty affairs in those days and soon I was off back to England." They didn't see much of one another until the end of the war, though Joe admits to occasionally breaking the rules to steal a night with Jane.

"We went into France with the D-Day landings and were stationed in Aramanche. The French seemed to resent us because we'd had to go to their aid. But soon we were in Holland. The Dutch were very friendly. You never gave a Dutchman anything that he didn't try to pay you back."

"One day we were told there were two German raiders around. Suddenly they were flying overhead very low. We were out in the open with nowhere to run. With machine gun fire raging all around, it was a case of heads down, bums up."

Having been delighted when the war started, Joe was just as pleased when it ended because he couldn't wait to get home to Scotland and to Jane, who had been working at an aircraft factory in Prestwick. Rita, their first child, was born in 1945, followed by John in 1947 and Joe Junior eight years later. When Joe was invited to rejoin 602 Squadron, which was reformed in 1946, Jane put her foot down. Instead he went back to working as a toolmaker at an engineering works in Ayr and later for Scottish Aviation at Prestwick. His younger son now works in Germany for British Aerospace.

Not that there have not been some exciting moments. In 1939 Joe became the penpal of the great Bing Crosby. They continued to correspond after the war and when Bing visited Ayrshire, he phoned Joe to invite him to play golf at Turnberry.

After Jane passed away in 1991, Joe lived with his daughter, a primary school teacher. But macular degeneration was robbing him of his sight and Rita also had health problems that made it increasingly difficult to care for her father.

"He started going to Erskine for respite care and every time he came back he seemed much perkier," says Rita. "One day he said 'I'd like to stay in Erskine for good but could you cope on your own?'. It was like an answer from God." He moved in during 2009 and to his utter delight found he was to be living in McKellar Ward, named after his old pal Archie, the Spitfire ace. "It was like being reunited."

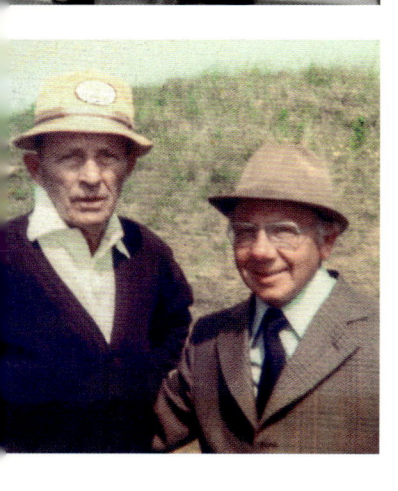

After the war, Joe returned to his job as a toolmaker

Joe with his famous penpal Bing Crosby at Turnberry.

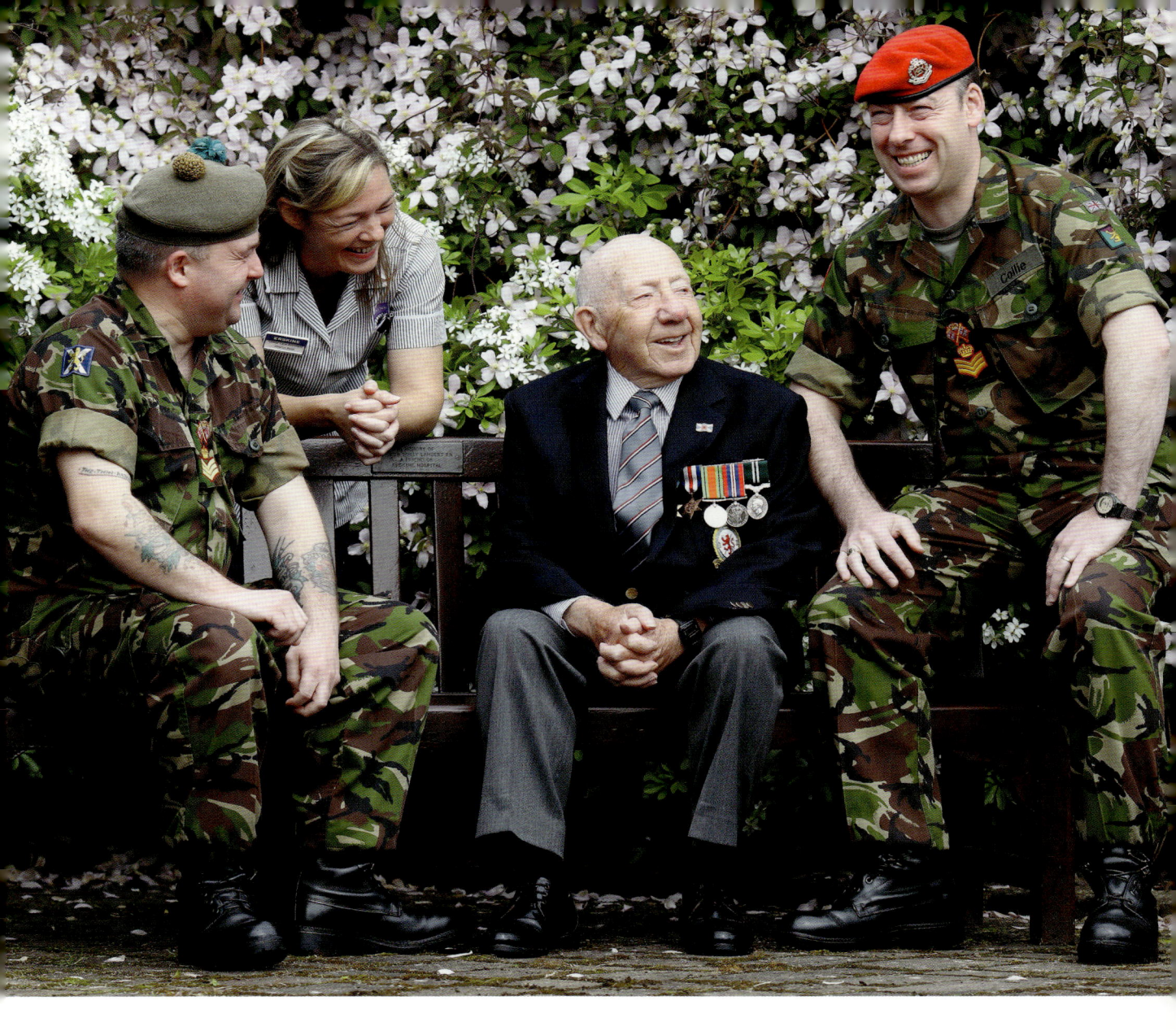

Erskine has given Joe a new lease of life. After the move he became a great fundraiser, appearing as the face of Erskine on the charity's "Support a Hero" leaflet. As he puts it: "When I came here I started living again, not just looking out of the window."

His bright room is filled with family photographs and pictures of his beloved planes. Despite his failing sight, his face lights up as he tells a story and there is a quiet dignity about this man. There is sadness too. Though Joe is delighted that the Spitfire hanging in Kelvingrove Museum is one of the most popular exhibits, today's visitors will never fly in one. And though he has tried to keep in touch with the 602 Squadron Museum in Glasgow and with his old comrades, with each passing year their ranks thin further. Only a small handful were there with him to witness the unveiling in 2013 of a granite memorial at Kelvingrove to celebrate 602's battle honours.

More than anything the story of Joe Parker is the story of the Spitfire. It was not merely the first all metal fighter plane. Thanks to the skills of men like Joe Parker and the courage and brilliance of men like Archie McKellar, the Spitfire has become a national icon and a reminder of a victorious past as Britain faces an uncertain future.

The face of Erskine: Joe has appeared in many photographs promoting and fundraising for Erskine.

Bill Anderson

"It took me a second or two to realise that here were Winston Churchill and Anthony Eden, returning from their meeting with Roosevelt and Stalin at Yalta."

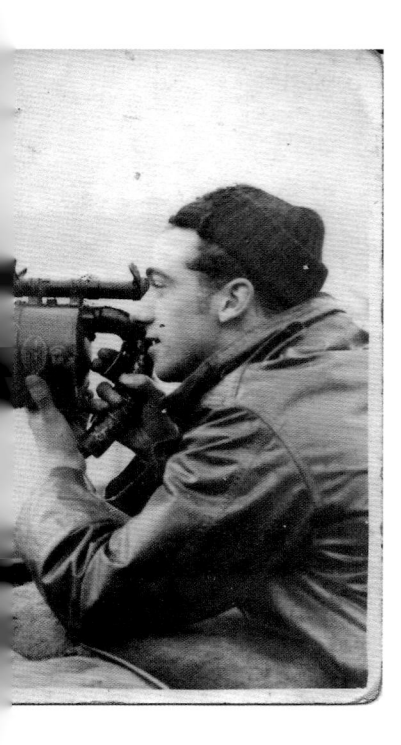

Bill on HMS Dunluce Castle with his Aldis lamp.

It is February 1945. The Second World War is drawing to a close, at least in Europe. Navy Signalman William Anderson from Maryhill is on a heavily-guarded dockside in the Crimea, attempting to stamp some heat into his freezing feet, when he spots two figures hurrying towards him through the darkness.

The older of the two is squat and burly; by contrast, the younger man is tall and debonair. The pair are deep in conversation and both have hats pulled down over their foreheads. "It took me a second or two to realise that here were Winston Churchill and Anthony Eden, returning from their meeting with Roosevelt and Stalin at Yalta," says Bill.

They need a lamp to show them the way along the jetty to the launch that will take them out to their accommodation on board the SS Franconia anchored in the bay, and a lamp is just what Bill is holding. Without a second thought he steps forward to help Britain's wartime leader and his Foreign Secretary to find their way. Seven decades later Bill Anderson, now a resident of Erskine Glasgow, recalls his walk-on role in world history as if it was yesterday. No wonder he's known as "the Yalta man."

It was no ordinary lamp that Bill was holding that night but an Aldis lamp, pioneered by the Royal Navy in the late 19th century to deliver signals at sea, usually using Morse code. (The pulses are produced by using a pressure switch to open and close a shutter in front of the lens.) When he had been conscripted in June 1941, the recruiting officer asked 19-year-old Bill his occupation. "When I said I worked for the GPO, he said: 'Right, communications for you, lad' and that's how I landed in the navy as a signalman."

Bill had left North Kelvinside Secondary at 14 to become a telegram boy. "I did well at Dunard St Primary and loved both maths and English. I believe I got the top mark in my "qualy" but I left school at 14 after taking an exam to get into the GPO." Besides, at home, there was a looming problem. Bill's dad, James, never really recovered from the First World War.

"I remember him standing at the sink to wash and seeing his hands shaking, though he was still quite young." Soon he was unable to work.

James had been the fifth of eight children of a bookbinder. Born in 1894, he grew up in a room and kitchen in Govan, later moving to St George's Cross. Strikingly handsome and a bit of a dandy, he had worked as an electrical engineer and served in the Territorial Army before volunteering for the 1/5th (City of Glasgow) Battalion of the Highland Light Infantry after the outbreak of WW1. He survived the horrors of Gallipoli and fought elsewhere in the Middle East. By the time he was demobbed in February 1919, he was a Company Sergeant Major. But, as Bill puts it: "Afterwards he wasn't the same man who had gone away."

James married his sweetheart, Lizzie McDonald, in 1920 and they settled down in Northpark St, beside Firhill Stadium, but Bill, born the following year, would be their only child. The only surviving childhood photo shows a skinny, cheery, bright-eyed 8-year-old Bill playing in his backcourt with two pals.

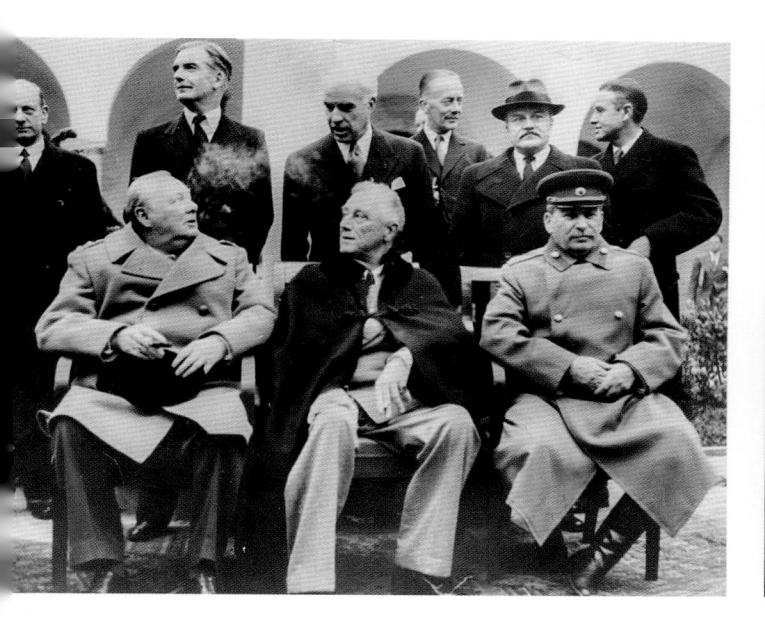

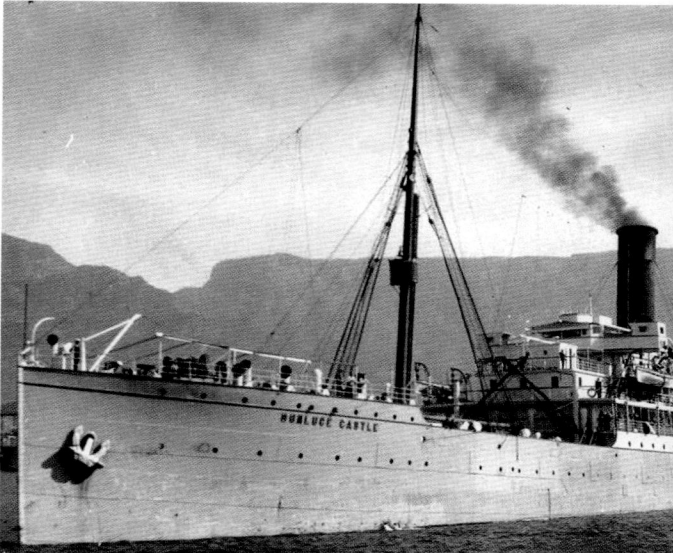

"Dad worked for Henderson's in Sauchiehall St but he was never very healthy and my wonderful mother had to work very hard to keep us going. She did cleaning jobs and anything she could get to make a few shillings."

Gradually his father began to lose control of his muscles and around the outbreak of the Second World War he was admitted to what was then known as the Princes Louise Hospital for Ex-Servicemen at Erskine. Today Bill treasures a single faded photograph of himself with his dad, taken in the hospital grounds in 1940.

"I would go down to Old Kilpatrick by bus, then across on a big ferry that was driven by chains. At first Dad was in one of the huts in the grounds. One day in March 1941 my bus took a detour because the normal route was covered in rubble and debris from the German bombing of Clydebank and hundreds of people had been killed. Further up, two oil tanks were still on fire with black smoke going up into the sky. It was shocking to realise what the Germans could do to your country. Dad and the other patients heard the whole thing. It must have been a terrifying experience for them."

Two months later Bill was in the uniform of a Royal Navy Signalman. After training at HMS Ganges in Ipswich and Highnam Court near Gloucester, he was dispatched to Orkney with the name HMS Dunluce Castle across his hatband. (By an odd coincidence, the same ship had ferried troops into Gallipoli in 1915.) Bill would spend most of the war in Lyness on the island of Hoy overlooking Scapa Flow. The Dunluce Castle was the main mail-sorting depot for the fleet and would sometimes provide a few days' welcome fresh air for submarine crews passing through the area. It was also used to accommodate survivors from the Arctic convoys. Bill became proficient at not only Morse code but also semaphore.

"I was there for about three years. I played football and table-tennis for the ship's team and when a whole lot of servicewomen appeared, there were Saturday night dances at the big NAAFI club onshore. I was dance-mad in those days."

In fact, he was to meet Nancy, the love of his life, on the dance floor, though it was not in Orkney but Glasgow. "Whenever I got a few days' leave, I'd head home even though the ferry journey across the Pentland Firth could be pretty hairy, especially in an ancient steamer called the St Ninian. I always wanted to get home, not only to visit Dad at Erskine but also

Winston Churchill, Franklin D. Roosevelt and Joseph Stalin at the Yalta Conference. Foreign Secretary Anthony Eden stands behind the Prime Minister.

HMS Dunluce Castle.

spend a few days in the Glasgow dance halls. The Berkeley, the Locarno, the Dennistoun Palais, the Albert. I loved them all. I met Nancy at a dance at Green's Playhouse one Wednesday. She mentioned she was going to a tea dance at the Plaza in Eglinton Toll on the Saturday, so of course I went, hoping to see her. It was instant love. We just clicked. We ended up back at the Playhouse on one of the Golden Divans in the cinema there." (These were double-width seats on the lower balcony, much favoured by courting couples, despite their exorbitant price of nine shillings – Bill's weekly earnings were just ten shillings and sixpence at the time.)

In early 1945 he was told to report to the SS Franconia in Liverpool for a special mission. Winston Churchill was to meet US President Franklin Roosevelt and Russian leader Josef Stalin in the Crimea to put together their final strategy for winning the war and shaping the future of Europe.

Bill remembers sailing through the Dardanelles, where his father had fought the Turks three decades before. The Franconia was a commandeered Cunard luxury liner, and onboard accommodation had been prepared in anticipation of using it for the conference itself. In the event the Russians had hastily spruced up (and, as it turned out, probably bugged) two palaces in Yalta for use by the British and American delegations. The Franconia anchored off Sevastopol from where the British delegation was taken across the Crimean peninsula by car.

Today historians argue about the significance of the accord reached at Yalta between the three great powers and whether Britain and the US were outmanoeuvred by Stalin but there is no doubt that at the time it was seen as the linchpin for a settlement that would not only end the war in Europe but also create a sustainable peace.

That sense of a historic achievement comes across powerfully in the speech Anthony Eden made before Bill and the rest of the Franconia's crew on February 14 1945 in which he thanked them for their help: "Perhaps history will say that the Crimea Conference did two things. It perfected the measures for the final defeat of Germany and it made some contribution to keeping that peace once victory is won. Our ability to keep the peace depends on the ability of the Great Three Powers – the United States, the British Commonwealth and Empire and Soviet Russia – to work together. If they can work together, peace is possible, maybe probable, for a generation. If they cannot work together it is hard to see any future but perplexity, suffering and war. It is as simple as that." (Bill's dog-eared and fading copy of the speech, given to him on the Franconia, still lies in his bottom drawer at Erskine.)

Churchill's stay on the Franconia was a brief one, before being whisked away to more talks in the Middle East but he too left a statement of thanks to the crew. In particular he says: "You carried here and accommodated signal personnel and communications, which have made it possible for me and my advisers to keep in constant touch with the progress of the war and to keep His Majesty's Government in London informed of the progress of the Conference." Everyone aboard should be proud of playing their part in such an historic event, he says, adding the request that the captain should "splice the mainbrace tonight."

Bill can't recall whether he actually received this extra rum ration. Besides, by now he had another major event on his mind. "We never got engaged but I'd said to Nancy that we would get married the next time I got home. I'd been to Jackson's and had a suit made." And so, one month after Yalta, Bill walked down the aisle in Glasgow with his Nancy on his arm. "I had to go back to my ship afterwards but soon I got my demob number and when

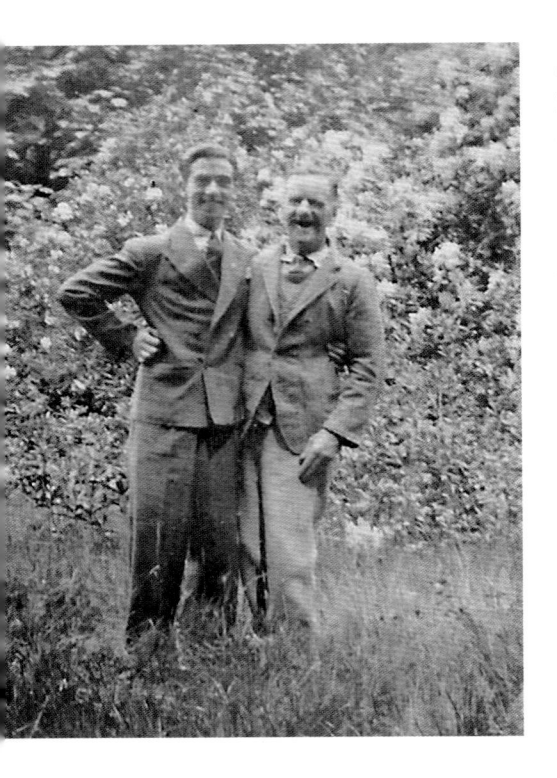

Bill and his dad James at Erskine in 1940.

the number came up I went to Edinburgh to collect a soft hat, a suit and a waterproof coat. I couldn't get home quick enough."

Though they had exchanged letters constantly, Bill and Nancy had spent fewer than 40 days together between meeting and marriage. Yet, like so many of those hasty wartime couplings, their marriage was a long and happy one. If it had a soundtrack, it was the music of Frank Sinatra and Dean Martin, which they both adored.

Bill went back to the GPO and worked for a time as a postman in the Firhill area. He and Nancy also managed to get a flat on Firhill Road. Having been born in the year that Partick Thistle beat Rangers to take the Scottish Cup, Bill has always had a weakness for the Jags, which can be a painful condition: "You'd come back from a match and say 'They were terrible. I'm never going back' but then the next week when you heard the 'thump, thump' of footsteps heading for the ground, you'd go back to see if they'd improved!"

At this time Bill's dad James was still at Erskine but his condition was deteriorating: "Eventually he was moved from the huts into the main house and on to a ward for paraplegics. Today I think he would have been diagnosed as having Parkinson's. The man in the next bed couldn't move at all and I remember the nurse would light a cigarette for him and he would smoke in his bed with his head to one side, letting the ash fall on to a small tray." James passed away at Erskine in 1951. Erskine's records show the cause of death as "sleepy sickness."

By then Bill and Nancy's first child, Isabel, was aged four and her sister Carole came along the next year. Bill was soon working for British Telecom. The family later moved to Cadder and Bill gave up playing football for his works team in favour of golf. He was a member at Windyhill near Bearsden. Bill and Nancy continued to love ballroom dancing. There's a great photo of them tripping the light fantastic at Butlin's in Ayr. Bill has always had a sharp mind and developed a passion for newspaper competitions. This paid off handsomely when he won a £2,500 diamond ring from the Evening Times. He had never bought Nancy an engagement ring so it was a question of better late (60 years late) than never.

By this time Bill had retired and the couple were enjoying a great life, travelling all over the world as far as South Africa and Hawaii. On cruises Bill liked to wear whites and a sailor's hat. As a result he was often mistaken for a member of the crew.

In later life Bill and Nancy had taken up bowling and it was while walking home from a bowling tie in October 2005 that Nancy fell in the street and died shortly afterwards. Bill still finds it hard to talk about this, though he continued bowling until he was 90 and even after coming to live at Erskine continued to participate in tea dances.

With Isabel and Carole now living in South Africa and Canada with their families, Bill had found living alone very tough. "I was down in the dumps but my daughters urged me to come to Erskine and I moved here in 2012. I love it because it gives me both freedom and support. It's a very sociable place" Since a recent fall, he needs to use a wheelchair and requires more care but Erskine is there to offer that.

Bill turned 94 in 2015. These days he likes nothing better than to think about his family – now swelled by four grandchildren and a great grandson – and all the snippets that have made his life such a rich tapestry. And although seven decades have slipped by since Signalman William Anderson stood on that dockside in the Crimea, clutching his Aldis lamp, in the minds of everyone who knows him, he will always be "the Yalta man."

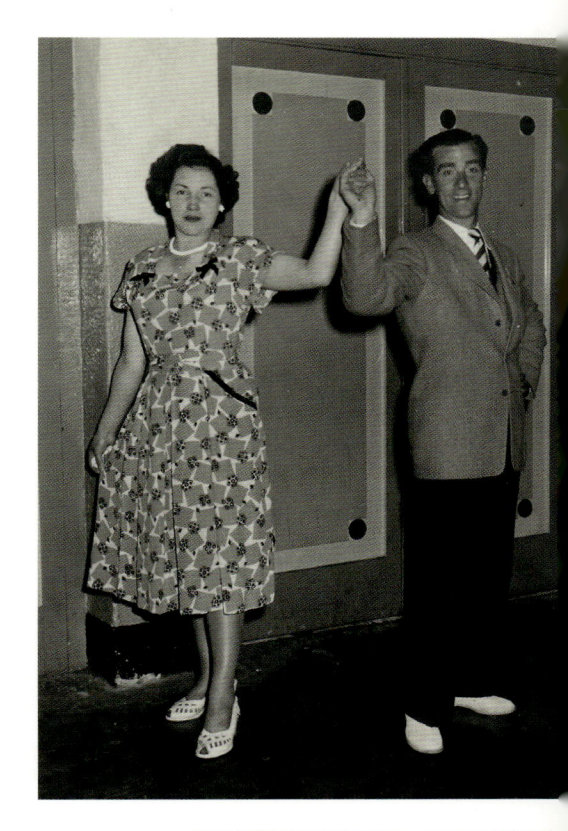

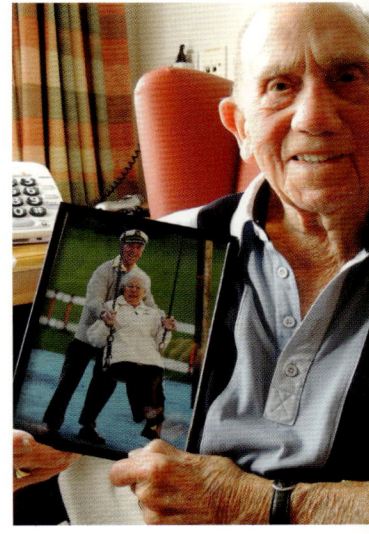

Bill and Nancy dancing at Butlin's in Ayr.

At home in Erskine with a picture of Nancy.

Jack Harrison & Alex Lees

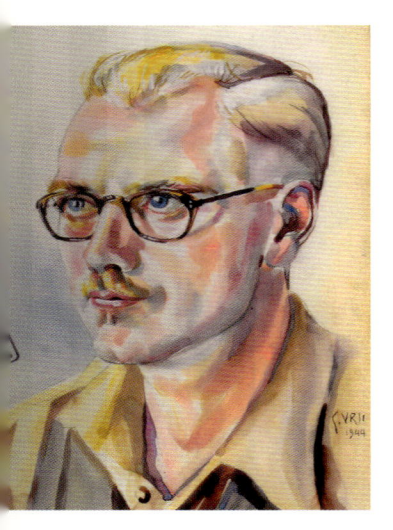

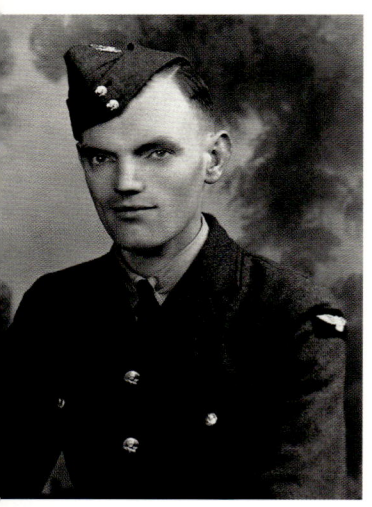

"Being in charge of the garden, I was able to dig a trench and disguise the sand by scattering it in the bottom and planting radishes, cress and tomatoes." Alex Lees

Will we ever cease to be intrigued by the Great Escape? The brave and extraordinarily tenacious (if ultimately largely unsuccessful) attempt by Allied prisoners-of-war to escape from the Luftwaffe-run camp Stalag Luft III has been celebrated in a succession of books and, of course, the celebrated 1963 Hollywood film.

Stalag Luft III was built in the German province of Lower Silesia near the town of Sagan (today known as Zagan) in Poland), 100 miles from Berlin and deliberately sited on sand to make tunnelling difficult.

The mass break-out took place on Friday, March 24, 1944. The driving force behind the ambitious plan was Roger Bushell, a charismatic Squadron Leader, the son of a South African mining engineer, who, as 'Big X', masterminded the digging of the three tunnels codenamed Tom, Dick and Harry 30ft below. (Bushell was played by Richard Attenborough in John Sturges' film.)

The prison camp had a number of design features that made escape extremely difficult. The huts housing the prisoners were raised approximately two feet off the ground to make it easier for guards to detect tunnelling, the camp was constructed on land with a very sandy subsoil, which could easily be detected on the grey surface and meant tunnels were liable to collapse. In addition, microphones were placed around the perimeter of the camp to detect any sounds of digging.

The stories of Alex Lees and Jack Harrison are particularly fascinating. Lees helped dispose of the huge quantities of sand from the clandestine digging operation. Harrison, who was a runner to Bushell, was waiting his turn to escape via Harry, the only remaining viable tunnel. Once outside, he was to pose as a Hungarian electrician in the employ of a German firm. He never got his chance. However, 76 men managed to escape before the alarm was raised.

Lees wrote a vivid memoir about his experiences, entitled Before It's Too Late. He died on April 22, 2009, and Jack Harrison on June 4 the following year, their parts in the Great Escape celebrated in numerous obituaries.

Alex Lees was born in Manchester in July 1911 but his family returned to Scotland when he was 11 and he was educated at Paisley's Camphill High School. He worked for a number of insurance companies in Glasgow before joining the Royal Army Service Corps in 1940. He was captured by the Germans 1941 and held in several POW camps before Stalag Luft III, which had opened early in 1942.

Jack Harrison, from Glasgow, was a classics teacher at Dornoch Academy in Sutherland when he was called up and joined the RAF as a pilot. His first mission, in a Lockheed Ventura aircraft in November 1942, was to bomb German supply ships at the Dutch port of Den Helder. Because his compass had not been calibrated properly, he ended up 12 miles off

Top: Alex Lees' self portrait.

Above: Jack Harrison in his RAF uniform.

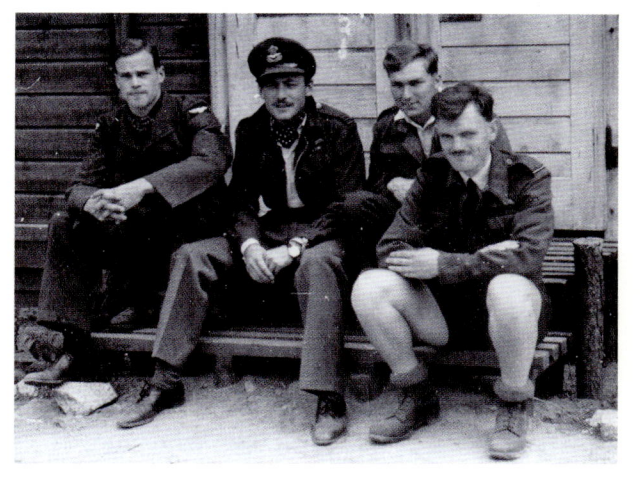

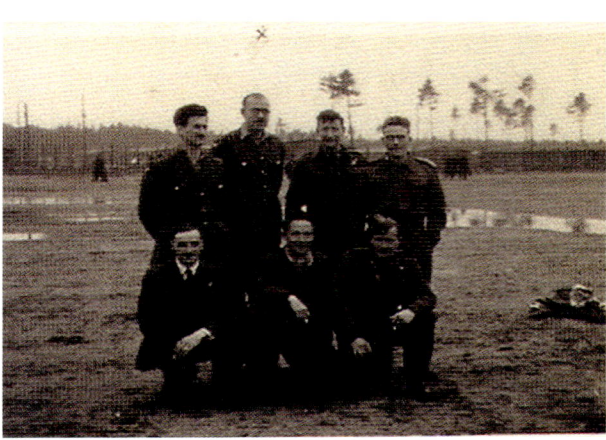

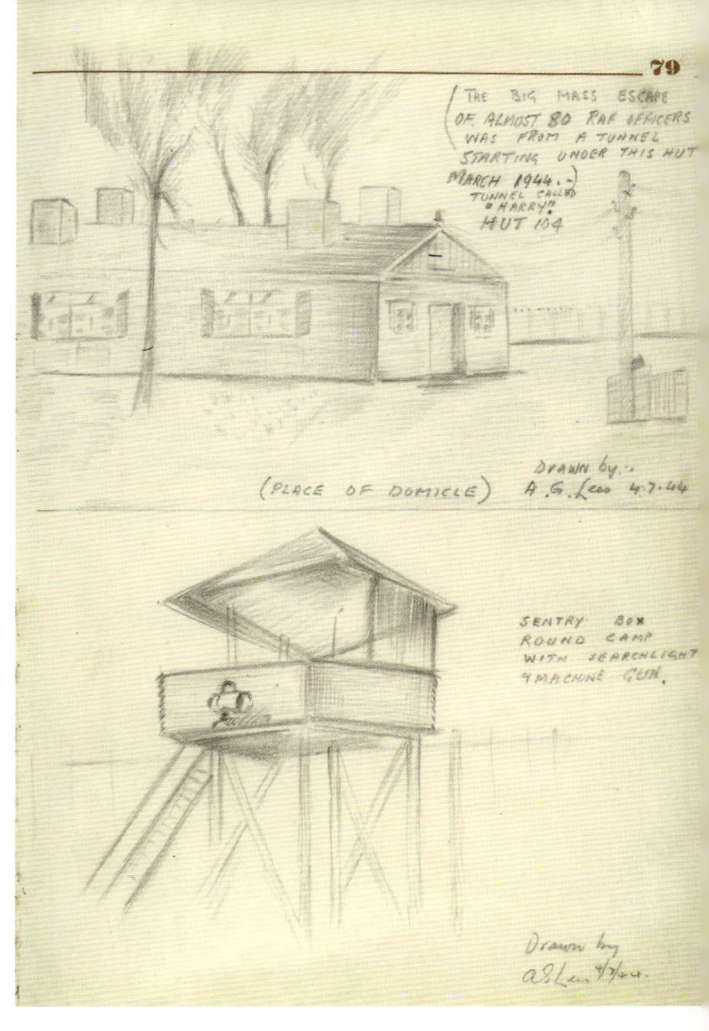

course, flying over water. The constant flak from the Germans from the ground eventually brought down the plane down.

"I was flying six feet above the beach at this point – that's fine when you're over land, but it's a different story over water," he would say, years later. "I started to weave to avoid the flak and did a slight turn and put my wing in the water. The sea came rushing over the top of the cockpit and we were going down, which was a worry for me as I couldn't swim. Three of us got out."

They could not find their fourth colleague, who had been injured during the attack. The group were picked up by fishermen but their rescue was shortlived. Before long they found themselves in enemy hands. He was transferred to Stalag Luft III.

Within the confines of this PoW camp, surrounded by pine trees, the resolve to outwit the Germans and enable a mass break-out to take place came from Sqdn Ldr Roger Bushell. He set in train the elaborate plan not only to dig the three tunnels but also to provide the escapees with civilian clothes and provide them with the money, rations, briefcases and ID cards that would be vital should they make it out of the camp.

Lees' task was to look after a garden outside his hut. In a 2007 interview, he recalled: "The Germans knew tunnels had been excavated at other camps, so we had to be very careful in disposing of the sand. I transported the sand from the digging site to the garden in Red Cross boxes.

"Being in charge of the garden, I was able to dig a trench and disguise the sand by scattering it in the bottom and planting radishes, cress and tomatoes." The German guards

Top left: Jack Harrison (far right) with fellow POWs at Stalag Luft III.

Alex Lees (2nd right top row) with fellow servicemen.

Above: Alex Lees' drawing of Hut 104 at Stalag Luft III.

Jack Harrison & Albert Lees 45

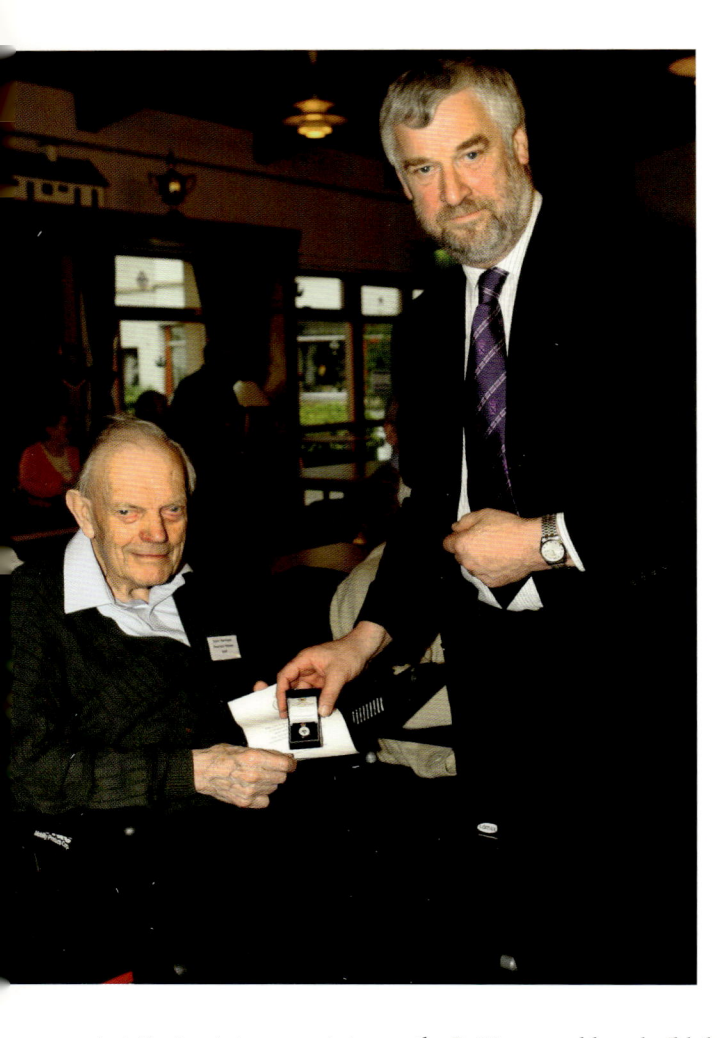

Jack Harrison being presented with his Veterans Badge by The Right Honourable Alex Fergusson MSP in The Erskine Home, Bishopton on 3rd July 2008.

would sometimes admire his efforts, little suspecting that his vegetables were an elaborate way to disguise what was going on nearby.

The prisoners' ingenuity knew no bounds: as Guy Walters relates in The Real Great Escape, two army kitbags were sewn together around a number of circular wooden frames 'to form an accordion-like tube, which was then mounted inside a long wooden box.' Leather flaps, reinforced with tin, were inserted into the tube; they acted as valves, opening and closing.

Wooden slats were removed from prisoners' beds in order to be used as pit-props. The prisoners also developed a simple but effective method of alerting the tunnellers whenever a German guard strayed too close.

As Lees recounted in 2007: "We had stooges following every guard who came into the camp. Someone would be reading a book, and they would suddenly put it down as a sign that someone was coming. It gave those working in the tunnel time to put back the hatch in the ground. The searches happened quite often. You could be sent out for two hours while they looked, which was quite scary. It didn't matter how much warning we tried to give those working in the tunnels, you never knew what they would find. It was a great risk."

The Germans knew that tunnelling was always a possibility. They installed special listening devices around the perimeter wires, designed to detect any signs of subterranean activity. Despite all these precautions, the PoWs were able to build their long tunnels without being detected.

A sign of the prisoners' remarkable success in keeping things hidden from the German guards was the extraordinary tally of items later found to have gone missing. This included 4000 bed boards, 90 double bunk beds, 635 mattresses, 192 bed covers, 161 pillow cases and 52 tables.

On March 24, hut 104 gradually filled up with the 200 men who would be escaping via 'Harry'. Dozens of men made good their escape but for one reason or another, the rate of escape gradually slowed down. When at 5am a German guard noticed movement in the woods, the game was up.

Lees had not been one of those chosen to be an escapee. "I wasn't eligible because it was for officers only," he later recalled. He had mixed feelings about this: on the one hand, he wanted to go, but on the other, he spoke no German. His role, instead, was to act as a decoy for one of the escapees. The plan was that he would take the bed of Flight Lieutenant Thompson. After the discovery of the escape, a German guard burst into the room, shouting at him, demanding he give his name. A swift check revealed that his photograph did not match that of Thompson. He was marched outside along with other prisoners. They had an anxious wait, assuming their last moments had come. After several hours shivering in freezing temperatures, however, they were allowed to return to their huts. Lees would later reflect that they owed their lives to the fact that Stalag Luft III was run by the Luftwaffe under the terms of the Geneva Convention; had the camp been run by the Gestapo, things

46 A Century Of Care: Erskine 1916 — 2016

might have been very different. Flt Lt Thompson himself was captured after just eight hours on the run.

Of the 76 escapees, just three made it to England. The others were recaptured and 23 returned to Stalag Luft III but the remaining 50, Bushell amongst them, were executed on the orders of Hitler. Lees knew several of them. Hitler's decision is regarded as constituting the single greatest war crime committed by Nazi Germany against British servicemen in the Second World War. At the Nuremberg trials, the execution of the 50 was one of the many subjects on which Hermann Goering, head of the Luftwaffe, was questioned.

Lees was sent to another PoW camp, where he remained until the end of the war. When he returned home he resumed his career in insurance, eventually becoming life and pensions superintendent at the Commercial Union. He married Isobel in 1946 and they had two children, Colin and Patricia. After he was widowed, he was able to live out his final years at Erskine. He wrote his evocative memoir and often toured schools to promote the work done by Erskine

For Jack Harrison, "it was a blessing in disguise I never made it through as most were shot, including Roger Bushell. But the main purpose wasn't just to escape. It was to outfox the Germans. It was a huge moral victory."

He was able after hostilities ceased to return home to his wife, Jean, whom he had married in 1940. He resumed his teaching career and ended as director of education at Bute County Council until retiring in 1975. He took up marathon running in his 70s to raise money for charity.

As fate would have it, he and Alex Lees were unaware of each other until both were in their nineties. Although they had been in the same camp, at its height it had held almost 1000 prisoners. A neighbour of Harrison's from Rothesay visited Erskine and discovered that Lees had been at Stalag Luft III. The two veterans finally met in November 2006 to share their stories and memories.

Alex Lees died at the age of 97 in 2009. By then Jack Harrison had also moved to Erskine, where he lived for two-and-a half years before his death in June 2010, also at the age of 97. His son and daughter said that while others considered him a war hero, "to us he was much more than that. He was a family man first and foremost, as well as a church elder, Rotarian, scholar, traveller and athlete."

The Great Escape is now more than seven decades ago but is still commemorated. In March 2014 hundreds of people assembled in Zagan, Poland, to remember those who died. Air Vice Marshal Stuart Atha told them that The Great Escape was "an extraordinary chapter" in the history of the allied air forces "written by men with great courage and character."

He described the escapees as "an exceptional band of airmen whose bravery, ingenuity and resilient spirit set an example for all time. When first captured, they did not accept that for them the war was over. Far from it, they were not prisoners of war – they were prisoners at war. And through their activities, they opened another front that distracted and diluted enemy forces and demonstrated that no fence, no Stalag Luft, could contain allied airmen."

In his room in Erskine, Mr Lees, ever modest, insisted that he had only played a "small part" in the Great Escape. Small, perhaps, but important. The heroism shown by everyone involved in the Great Escape seemed to have stayed with him. "I must admit," he said a few years ago, "I think about it all the time."

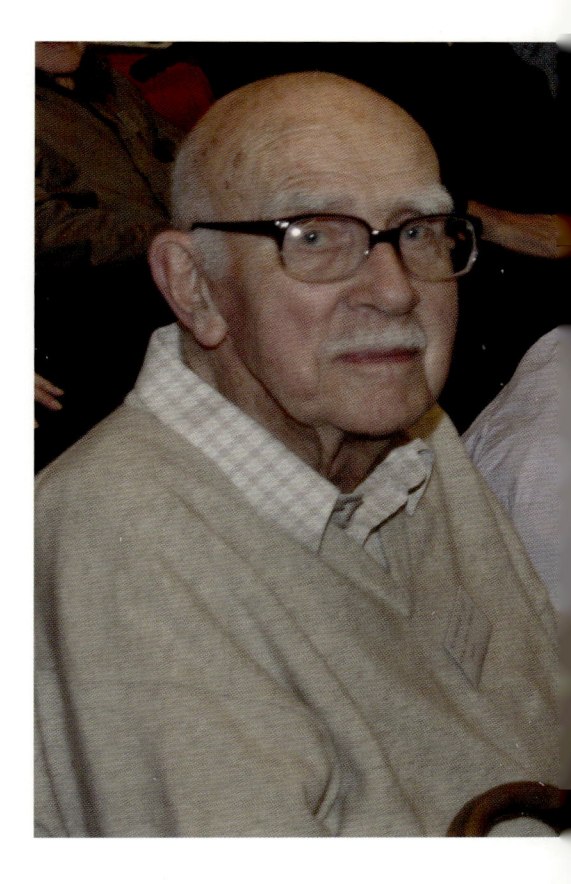

Alex Lees, The Erskine Home, Bishopton.

May McLean

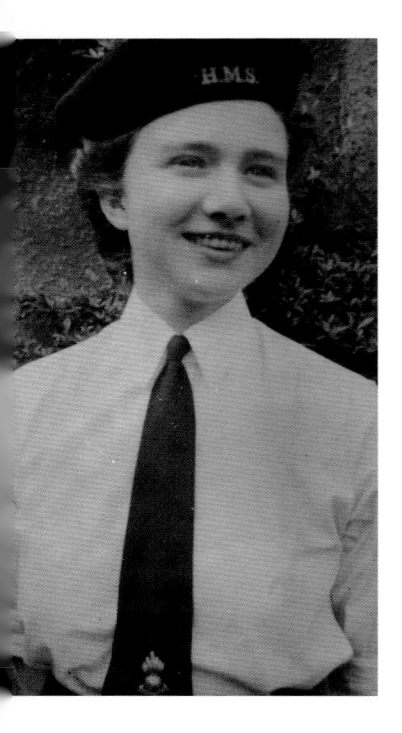

May in her WRNS uniform.

"Proud? I never ever thought about it. I just got on with the job in front of me and hoped I was doing it to the best of my ability."

Breaking the German Enigma Code during the Second World War did not merely shorten the war and save many lives. In the intervening decades the work done at Bletchley Park has developed a powerful hold on British collective consciousness. In an increasingly uncertain world and in a nation state unsure of what its role in the global order should be, Bletchley like other touchstone names – Spitfire, D-Day, Shackleton, Waterloo – embodies something we like to think of as reassuringly British: a potent mix of ingenuity, endeavour and pluck that can win through against the odds. These are the polished jewels in our common historical narrative.

What makes the Enigma story so compelling is not just the intellectual brilliance and painstaking attention to minute detail needed to crack a seemingly uncrackable code. It is also the way it brought disparate elements together. Part of the reason why Britain proved better at code cracking than Germany was the pooling of talent and resources between the Foreign Office, British Army, Royal Navy and the RAF. But it also represented a coming together at a human level. Until recently the story has been dominated by the handful of brilliant young men, predominantly Oxbridge and particularly the ill-fated Alan Turing. The caricature that personifies the WW2 intelligence gathering operation is an earnest youth in a tweed jacket with suede elbow patches. But as Tessa Dunlop observes in her book The Bletchley Girls, 7,000 of those who worked at Bletchley Park and its outstations were young women, mainly Wrens, handpicked for their ability to do tough monotonous work and keep their mouths shut. And that's exactly what they did. To such an extent that until very recently their contribution to the war effort has been almost entirely overlooked. One of these women is May McLean, who has lived at Erskine since 2010.

In April 2015 Tessa Dunlop's event about the women of Bletchley Park attracted a sell-out audience to Glasgow's Aye Write! festival, including May, who had read her book with interest. Delighted to find among the crowd no fewer than three living breathing "Bletchley Girls" (all in their 90s), Ms Dunlop invited them up on stage for a spontaneous question and answer session. Asked when she began her decoding work, May looked only briefly flummoxed before cracking into a huge smile: "They told us to forget everything and I seem to have succeeded!"

Then something unexpected happened. The packed predominantly female audience rose as one to its feet, cheering and clapping. Many had tears in their eyes. Afterwards dozens rushed forward to shake May's (immaculately manicured) hand. For a woman who has spent 65 years avoiding the subject of her war service, it was a surreal experience.

Until recently, if women were mentioned in connection with "BP", they were likely to have been posh girls whose fathers were senior military or foreign office personnel or brilliant girls who could do The Daily Telegraph crossword in no time, like Joan Clarke,

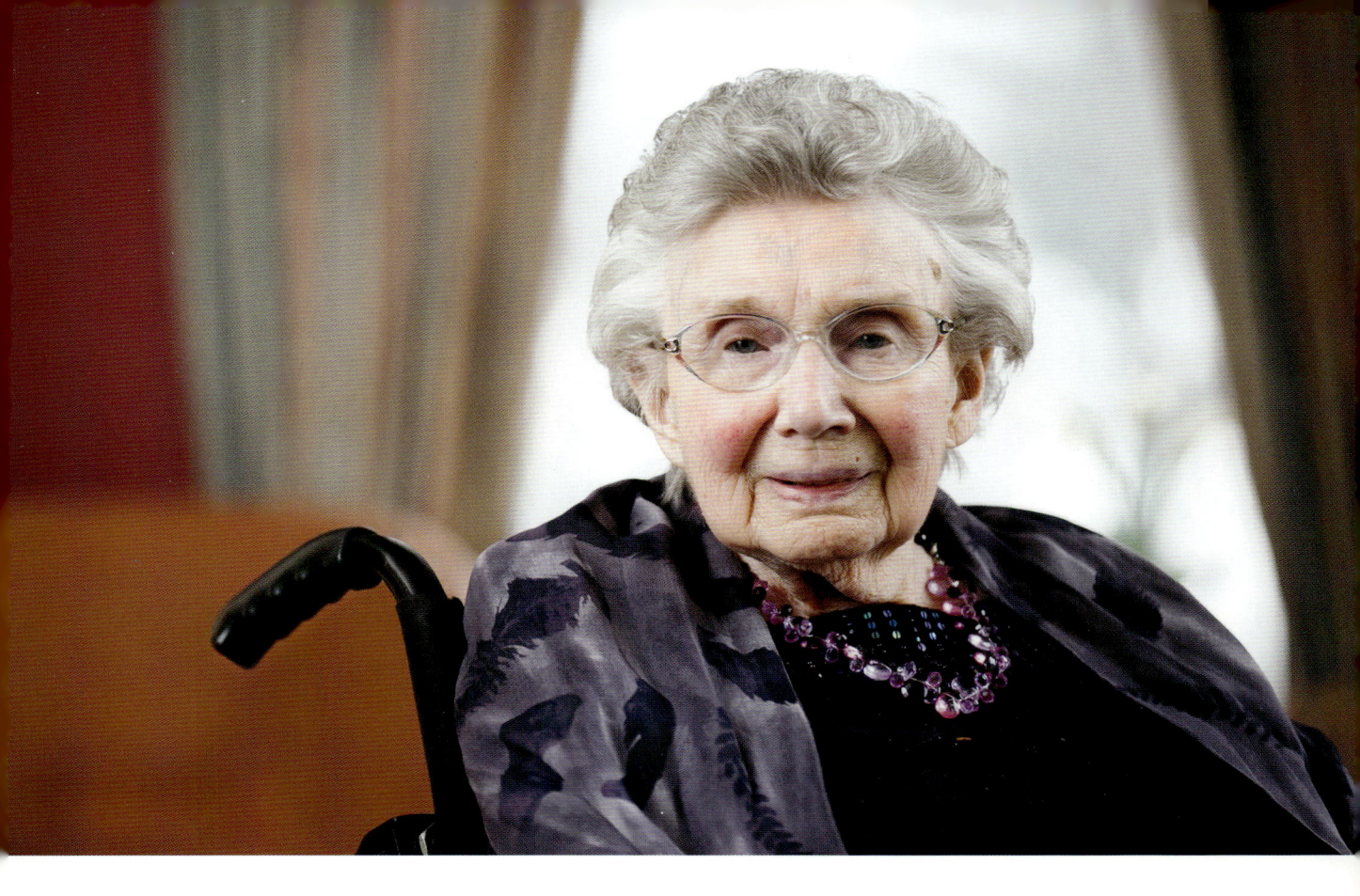

Life at Erskine has brought companionship and new activities.

played by Keira Knightley in the film *The Imitation Game*, the 2014 film about Nazi code breaking. But the vast majority of the women who worked in this field came from very ordinary backgrounds.

May was born Mary McKenzie McDowall on September 15 1922 in her grandparents' home in the Ibrox area of Glasgow. Her father George, one of ten children, was a cooper, as his own father had been. Her mother, Mary, a sewing machinist, came from Inverness. As an RNVR reservist, George had survived the disastrous Gallipoli campaign in 1915 and the couple had married in 1918, shortly before the end of the First World War.

A delightful portrait, taken around 1925, shows the young May looking slightly apprehensive and clasping a large doll. She would be the eldest of three, followed by the arrivals of Iain and then Valerie.

May began her education at the Charles Rennie Macintosh-designed, Scotland Street School, now a museum. "One of my first memories was falling off a swing. I had a compound fracture and spent six weeks in the old Yorkhill Hospital. I remember waving (with the other arm) to my relations out of the window because they weren't allowed inside."

It was a largely pleasant childhood. There were summer holidays in Kintyre and the Isle of Man and visits to her maternal grandparents in Inverness.

At Govan High her favourite subject was geography but if the young May pictured herself travelling the world, those dreams had to stay on hold for the meantime. Having secured her School Certificate, she took clerical jobs with Arthur & Co, a wholesale business in Queen St, and then the Clyde & Campbeltown Shipping Company in Robertson St.

"During the 1930s you weren't much aware of what was happening in Germany. There was no television and we weren't so well informed as today's youngsters. When war was declared, all the men thought it was going to be a great adventure. I didn't. I felt awful."

One day when the Luftwaffe showed up over Glasgow in 1941, May was in the city centre with her friend Dora. "The air raid siren went off and we were herded into the Savoy Cinema. Afterwards it took ages to get home because the trams were off. We found my mother and father and their friends had spent the evening sheltering under the dining table."

Initially May believed her job would be a reserved occupation. "When I realised I was likely to be called up, I went and joined the Wrens, because my father and brother had both been in the navy and because I didn't want to end up in a munitions factory. I was interviewed at a hotel in Glasgow and asked if I was interested in doing 'secret work'. We were told not to go blabbing about this to anyone, even our parents. I was sent to Leeds for training where there were lots of tests. They wanted to see if we were suitable and make sure we weren't flibbertigibbets!" She was also required to sign the Official Secrets Act, with the warning that revealing her work could be punishable by death.

Late in 1943 May was allocated to Stanmore in North London, one of the outstations serving the code-breaking centre at Bletchley Park. For the rest of the war her job was to work one of the many Bombe machines that Alan Turing and fellow cryptanalyst Gordon Welchman had developed in 1941 to crack the Enigma code, used by the Germans to send military reports and instructions.

With the Germans changing the code every 24 hours, cracking it became a daily race against time, with thousands of lives potentially hanging on success or failure.

"The machines were huge, as big as wardrobes. You had to stand on something to reach the top. They were full of wires and had rows of coloured discs on the front."

It was May's job to take down "cribs" (fragments of probable text, worked out by the decoders at Bletchley) and then set up the Bombes to test them by performing a chain of logical deductions. "We'd enter the letters and numbers and then set the machine going. It made a 'bumpity bump' sort of noise and when it stopped, we'd take down the letters and send them off. You were just a tiny cog in a big machine. You got bits of things that made sense when they were put together but it didn't mean a blooming thing to us." Though never told, May concluded that they were handling messages to and from German U-boats.

About 500 Wrens worked in shifts around the clock in huts behind a high fence guarded by armed marines and shuttled from their barracks by bus. "It could be dull and stressful but there was a tremendous camaraderie between us because they were the only ones you could talk to."

Despite the burden of regular drills and kit inspections, one advantage of Stanmore was that it was then at the end of the Bakerloo Line. "On days off we could get into the centre of London. I remember hiring a soap box to sit on while queuing for tickets for an opera or the theatre. We could only afford to sit in the gods but we didn't mind. And we had our own money, even if the pay was fairly meagre."

Her war did not end on VE Day in May 1945. Unexpectedly, May found herself among a handful of the girls from Stanmore selected to go to what was then Ceylon (Sri Lanka), one of the red blobs on the world map she remembered from geography lessons in Govan. Though she didn't realise it at the time, later she found that it had been to help decrypt Japanese military codes.

"I was excited. I had my inoculations and tropical uniform and off we went but the ship carrying us only got as far as North Africa when Hiroshima happened and the Japanese surrendered. So I never got to Sri Lanka, care of the British Government!" Typically, May omits to mention that during her service she was promoted to Leading Wren.

Back in Britain, after months spent helping decommission various naval stations, May received a prosaic letter from her employers re-instating her at the Clyde &

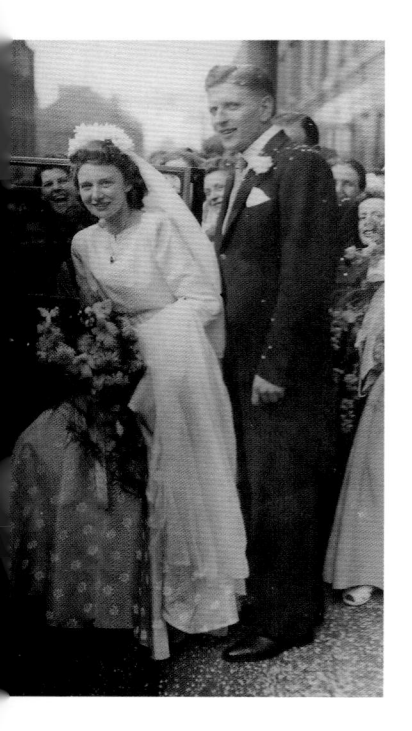

Setting off on married life: May and Neil McLean at their wedding in Glasgow in 1948.

Campbeltown Shipping Co at a salary of £160 a year. It was there that she met Neil McLean, a well-known amateur footballer who had played for Neilston Victoria and Dumbarton. The couple married in 1948.

During the war, as an acting staff sergeant in 530 Company of the Royal Army Service Corps, Neil had been awarded the Croix de Guerre with Palm from the Belgian government for the leadership he demonstrated by his cheerfulness and efficiency while under heavy mortar fire during the attack on Walcheren in November 1944. A newspaper report of the nuptials merely mentions that "The bride also served during the war for several years as Leading Wren in the Royal Navy."

Of course, May's lips were still sealed when it came to her war work. In fact, one regret she has is that her parents went to their graves without ever knowing that their daughter had played a small part in defeating the Germans.

Like most women who had served in the armed forces, May then buckled down to a rather humdrum domestic existence. She continued helping out with paperwork in what had now become a family-owned cooperage, and devoted herself to raising children Fiona and Iain. It must be said that "Mummy, what did you do in the war?" was hardly a common inquiry in the 1950s. Women's war service was not considered interesting or important, even if unscrambling Enigma and other German codes was every bit as important as beating the enemy on the ground in North Africa, France and the Burmese jungle. And those Bombe machines are now seen as the precursor of the information age.

Is she proud of her wartime service? "Proud? I never ever thought about it. I just got on with the job in front of me and hoped I was doing it to the best of my ability."

As May herself puts it: "We couldn't say anything for decades by which time we had forgotten most of it." In fact, it only dawned on her gradually that she was part of the Bletchley story at all. "Nobody ever mentioned Bletchley Park and I have still never been there. During the war I'd never heard of Alan Turing or the Enigma code." She was astonished when she was told that the work of the Bombe machines may have shortened the war by at least two years.

Neil McLean died in the late 1970s and May moved to Glenbarr near Campbeltown to live with her daughter Fiona and husband. Her son Iain, now steward at Machrihanish Golf Club, and his family were also nearby. May's granddaughter Kirsten was born in 1999.

"I had spent holidays in the area as a child and loved living in Kintyre. I didn't miss Glasgow one bit," says May. But in 2001 she suffered a serious stroke and shortly afterwards underwent a hip operation. Though she got back on her feet and made a good recovery, increasingly she became stranded at home. Her isolation was compounded by deep cutbacks in local authority social services.

Fiona says: "Respite care disappeared and we were down to three 15-minute visits a day. Mum was starting to ask: 'What's the point of living?'."

May moved to Erskine in April 2010. "On the day Mum moved in, three staff got down on their knees beside her wheelchair and told her: 'You have your family in Kintyre but now this is your home and we are your Erskine family.' The move has transformed her. She's always doing something. There are concerts and lots of activities like baking and food tasting. She's been on trips to places like the Falkirk Wheel and the Scottish Parliament." She especially enjoys her regular hairdo and manicure.

May has become a bit of an Erskine celebrity, photographed chatting with Prince Charles and Lorraine Kelly. Her daughter says simply: "If it wasn't for Erskine, Mum wouldn't be here by now."

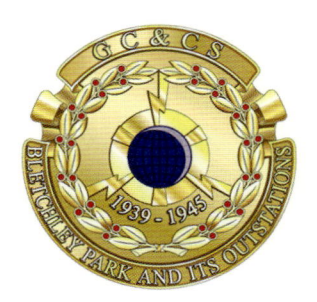

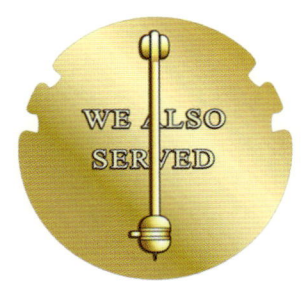

"I've never been one for medals and badges." says May McLean. But in 2015, following an application to GCHQ by her family, May was delighted to receive through the post a small parcel containing a Bletchley Park Commemorative Badge, issued to surviving veterans of the Government Code and Cypher School at Bletchley Park and its outstations. On the reverse side in small letters are the words: "WE ALSO SERVED."

May McLean 51

Joe 'Jock' Henry

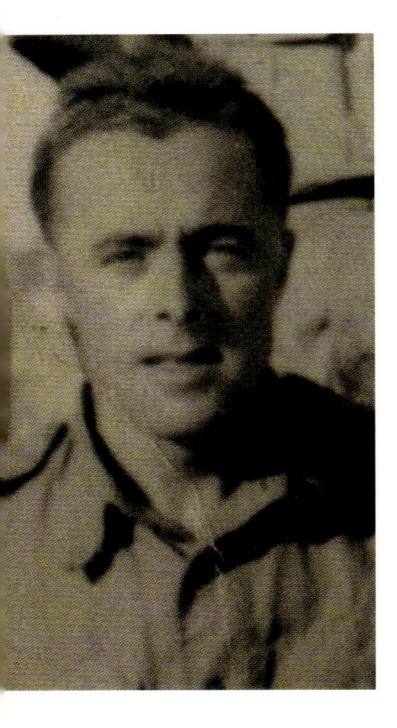

"It always comes back. It was a bad, bad time. But my real thought is about all the mates that I lost."

In December 1941 Joe Henry sailed from Greenock on the Empress of Australia, thinking that he and his colleagues were bound for the Middle East. But on the seventh of that month, the Japanese launched a surprise – and lethal – attack on the US naval base at Pearl Harbor, in Hawaii. Henry's destination now became the Far East, via Cape Town. Within a few months he would fall into the hands of the Japanese. He endured appalling treatment for more than three years before the war mercifully came to an end.

This is his story, as told by his son Hugh, the MSP for Renfrewshire South. He grew up at Erskine, where his parents lived from 1955 onwards. Erskine, Hugh and his siblings say, meant everything to Joe; it saved his life, and allowed him to live with dignity.

Joe Henry was born into a working-class family in the east end of Glasgow. Family circumstances meant that he had to leave school when he was just 14 – something that was fairly common at the time. He worked in the meat market at the Gallowgate, in a reserved occupation. He signed up in either 1939 or 1940, when he was still in his early twenties.

He was, recollects his son, Hugh, a very religious man. "I remember, when we were young, there was a point in the 1960s when it looked as though India and China were facing up to fight each other. He was panicking that this was all going to start again, and I remember he wanted us all to pray for peace."

Joe was a Lance corporal (number 241037) in the Royal Army Service Corps, attached to the 77th Heavy Anti-Aircraft Regiment of the Royal Artillery. He did his basic training in England, and set sail from Greenock in December 1941, arriving in Batavia (Jakarta), the capital of the Dutch East Indies, in February 1942. He was then moved to Surabaya to help guard the docks and airfields.

"Until they were captured," Hugh remembers, "I don't think they had fired a shot in anger. He worked in various places, making preparations, and then suddenly the Japanese swept in. There was no resistance."

The Americans, British, Dutch and Australians on Java surrendered on March 8. Joe was captured at Garut and taken to Tanjung Priok camp in Batavia (Jakarta). It was here that he helped to build a Church of England chapel. After a year, the Japanese transferred him to Surabaya, from where he was shipped to Ambon.

Joe was one of those prisoners on the Long March to Liang where he was involved in work on the airstrip and the docks. His family remember him saying that men such as Dennis Turner, Captain Bentley Taylor, Captain Smyth, an Australian named Bill Shepherd, and an Irishman by the name of Casey, all saved his life, at different points.

"He said the Japanese were pretty ruthless in their treatment of the prisoners. There were incidents when men were beheaded for not showing enough respect. Brutal beatings were a regular feature, let alone the terrible diets, and the work the men were put through. The Japanese showed them no mercy.

Joe Henry in Ceylon (now Sri Lanka) en route to Jakarta with the Royal Army Service Corps.

> **BUCKINGHAM PALACE**
>
> The Queen and I bid you a very warm welcome home.
>
> Through all the great trials and sufferings which you have undergone at the hands of the Japanese, you and your comrades have been constantly in our thoughts. We know from the accounts we have already received how heavy those sufferings have been. We know also that these have been endured by you with the highest courage.
>
> We mourn with you the deaths of so many of your gallant comrades.
>
> With all our hearts, we hope that your return from captivity will bring you and your families a full measure of happiness, which you may long enjoy together.
>
> *George R.I.*
>
> September 1945.

Letter from King George to returning POWs.

"When I was young, my dad taught us to count up to 20 in Japanese 'ichi, ni, san, shi, go …' and that was because they used to stand in line and call out their number. If you didn't respond, you got a beating."

Joe owed his life to several of his fellow prisoners, and his luck continued to hold out on November 29, 1943. Some 422 British servicemen and 127 Dutch PoWs were ordered into the hold of 4,645-ton Suez Maru bound for Java. Joe was supposed to join them, but at the last moment he was taken off the list. The Suez Maru was later torpedoed 330 km east of Java by the USS Bonefish. According to later accounts, many men drowned in the holds, although as many as 250 POWs were able to cling to flotsam. The minesweeper that had accompanied the Suez Maru collected Japanese survivors before opening fire on the men who were still in the sea. (It would be another seven years before the truth came out.) This episode, Hugh believes would come to weigh heavily on Joe – the acute sense of loss that so many of his friends had died, the thought that, 'there but for the Grace of God', he might have been on board the ship alongside them.

After some two years on Ambon, Joe returned to Java on the Taiwan Maru and taken to St Vincent's in Batavia. He was then moved to the Bicycle Camp and, lastly, to Bandoeng where, in August 1945, word filtered through that the war in the Pacific was finally over.

"I remember my dad saying that, at the end of the war, he didn't know if they were going to survive. The Japanese had told them to dig: they were digging their own graves. By that time, the Japanese realised they were losing and I think they were starting to massacre Allied prisoners. I remember him saying that he got up one day and the Japanese had disappeared. It was only later they found out that the bomb had been dropped." Hiroshima had been destroyed by an atomic bomb on August 6, three days later, it was the turn of Nagasaki.

"My dad always said that if it hadn't been for that, they would probably be dead. He never used it to say that you should glorify or justify nuclear weapons, or devastation on that scale: it was just a simple statement, that had that not happened, they would have been dead. It's quite a sobering comment."

Joe got word that the war was coming to an end from a fellow PoW, one Laurens van der Post, an Afrikaner who was serving with the British Army and had himself been a prisoner of the Japanese since April 1942. "Van der Post, who was in the same camp as my dad, had managed to get access to a radio, and he was able to tell him the news," says Hugh.

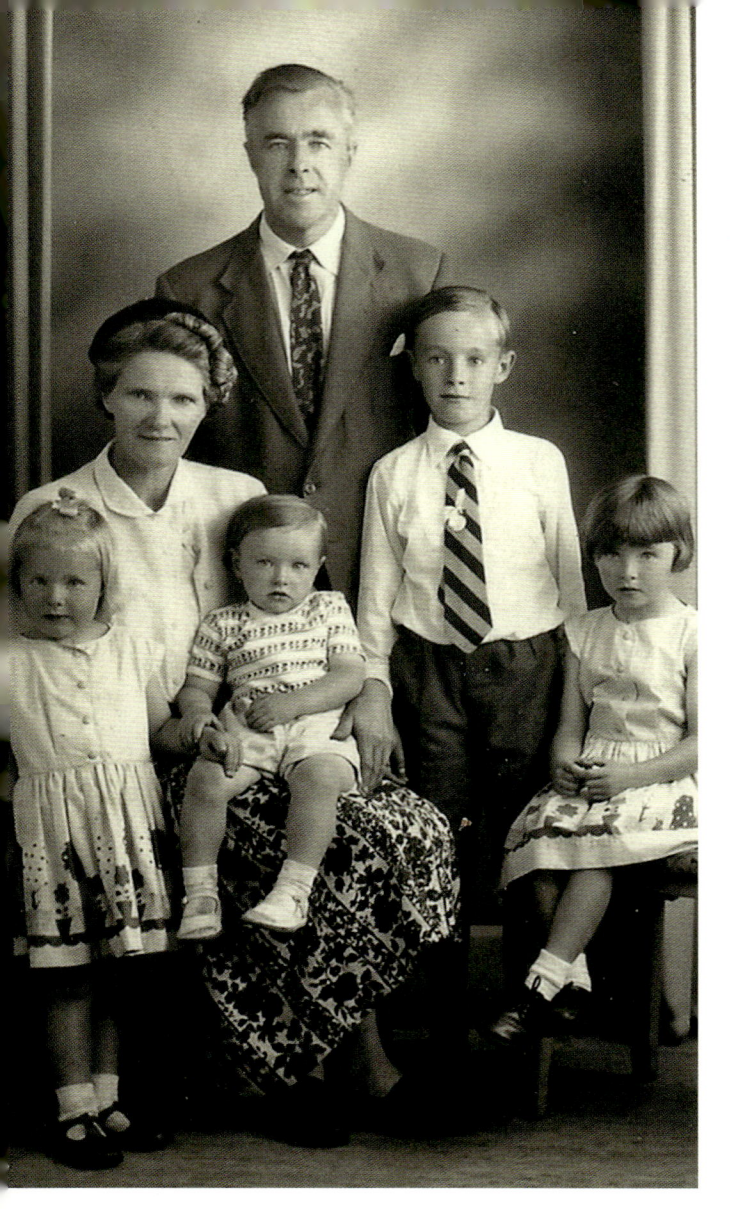

Joe and Mary Henry, with children (left to right) Patsy, Joseph, Hugh and Marian at Erskine in the 1950s.

The Japanese finally surrendered on August 14. The war in the Pacific was at an end.

Joe had suffered terribly. He was afflicted with beriberi, dysentery and malaria. He weighed just four and a half stones.

"The war obviously had a searing effect on him," says Hugh. "I don't know how I would have coped. I suppose his strong faith helped him through. I don't know how he might have coped otherwise with all of that."

The malaria would often come back in the years after the war. "When you're a child," reflects Hugh, "it's quite a frightening experience. The sweat would be pouring off him, the fevers … and I suppose there was also the memory of the horrors he'd witnessed. In those days there was no such thing as post-traumatic stress disorder. You just had to deal with it. He would shout out sometimes, he would have nightmares. He must have remembered what he had endured and also what had happened to his mates."

Indeed, Joe himself spoke about this, in August 1995, on the occasion of the 50th anniversary of VJ Day. Interviewed by STV's John Mackay, he said: "I had a lot of that –

bad dreams and whatnot, waking up with shudders. And that went on for quite a while. And it still happens. The likes of maybe today we're talking about it. Maybe tonight I'll have a wee setback … It always comes back. It was a bad, bad time. But that's my real thought – mates that I lost."

In the early 1970s, Joe and some of his fellow PoWs were called in for medical treatment: it was discovered that they all had tropical worms growing within them – another legacy of their time in the prison camps. There was yet another: the combination of poor diet, the constant reflection of strong sunlight off white sands, and being forced to stare at the midday sun on pain of being bayoneted, had damaged Joe's eyesight. He was in fact classified as blind, and in the last 20 years of his life he had to wear thick, goggle-type glasses so that he could read. But Hugh remembers something else: when he was young, his father was one of the few ex-servicemen in that circle who still had all four of his limbs. Another dad had lost both legs as he parachuted into Arnhem. Others had lost a leg or an arm or both while serving their country.

Joe had initially returned to the east end of Glasgow and settled down, married Mary, and began raising a family. Home was, at first, digs in Mauckinfauld Road, in Tollcross, which is where Hugh spent his first few years. In time, Joe and Mary were able to get a home within Erskine. What a difference it made: three bedrooms, an inside toilet complete with bath, and a back garden. "What a wonderful environment in which to bring up a family, Hugh reflects now, "especially after everything that all these guys had been through." He was able to talk to former servicemen who had endured similar experiences. It was almost as if they were part of their own Band of Brothers.

Joe lived at Erskine from 1955 until 2007, when he died, aged 91. "That was astonishing," his son says now, "when you think of everything that he had been through. How the heck did he manage to live for so long?

"When we were growing up, my mum was the strong one. She had to be. There were times when my dad wasn't able to work. In those early years, until the war pension improved, they were quite poor. My mum, when she was able to, used to take cleaning jobs in other people's houses in Bishopton, just to get a few bob to feed and clothe her four children. She also had to cope with my dad's frequent periods of ill-health. And yet, in the end, he outlived her."

Hugh can't forget these years he spent in the rural setting of Erskine. The place, he says, "helped my dad and the others to slowly reconcile themselves to what had happened during the war. It enabled them to get back into the routine of a normal life again. There was a great community spirit, too, and a lot of kids there who were within the same age range. For children Erskine was a wonderful, happy and safe environment. For our parents it was a place to rebuild shattered lives and overcome the pain and horrors of war. Erskine was a godsend for my dad and the other disabled ex-servicemen. It was ahead of its time. It was absolutely ahead of its time."

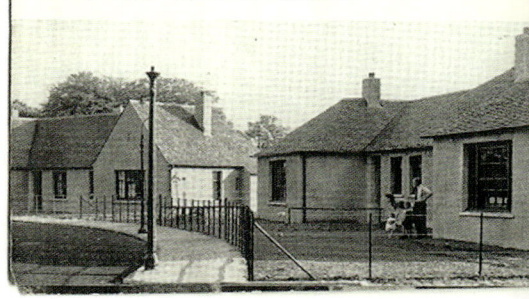

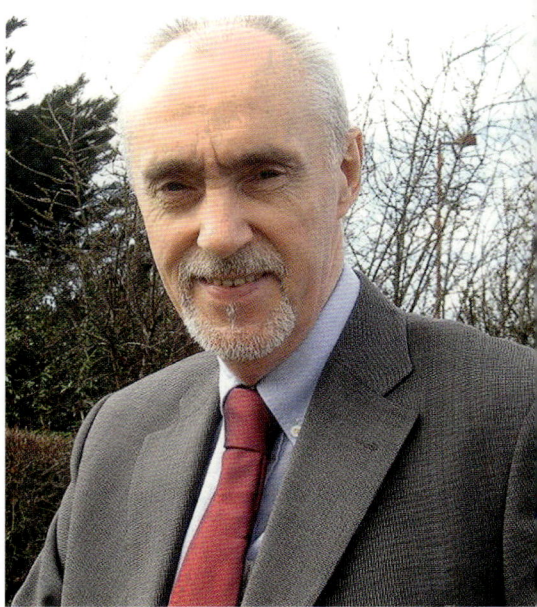

Top: Extract from an Erskine leaflet from the late 1950s showing the Henry family outside their veterans' cottage.

Above: Hugh Henry MSP, who spent a happy childhood at Erskine.

Joe Henry **55**

Maureen Lundie

"I wanted the patients at Erskine to realise that matrons are not all battleaxes. Some men will be patients for 30 or 40 years and they must not be made to feel institutionalised for life."

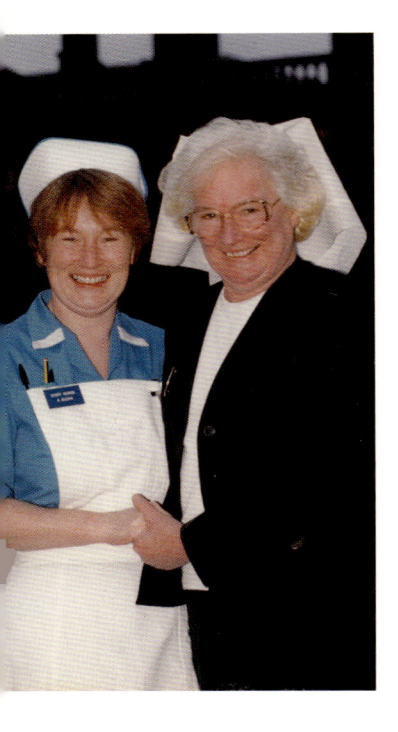

Like mother, like daughter. Maureen congratulates daughter Anne on qualifying as a nurse.

From the appointment of Miss A C Douglas in 1916, the matron was a pivotal figure in the success of Erskine Hospital. In 1977, Maureen Lundie, succeeded Mary Cameron, who had held the post for the previous 13 years. Creating a family atmosphere in a hospital which was also home to the majority of her patients had been central from the beginning but no matron would put it into effect quite as literally as Mrs Lundie, who moved into the matron's quarters in the Mansion House with her husband Peter and their six children, aged from 18 to six. "We were hospital brats," Anne, the eldest of the siblings, says cheerfully. "My mother had previously been the night duty nursing officer at Ruchill Hospital in Glasgow and we lived in a large, old house in the hospital grounds, so we were used to being around hospitals."

Maureen Lundie's guiding principle was to ensure everyone co-operated with each other. "It's just a question of knowing how to handle each person according to his particular temperament or needs. One thing above all everyone on the staff must remember is that Erskine is not just a hospital to most of the men here, it is their permanent home. Some men will be patients for 30 or 40 years and they must not be made to feel institutionalised for life."

In the late 1970s, however, the hospital was faced with a severe financial crisis. Running costs had escalated to reach £1m a year due to a combination of inflation, a spike in the price of oil for heating and a sharp increase in nurses' wages. To make ends meet, it had been necessary to liquidate some investments and take out a bank loan. At the annual meeting of the executive committee in 1978, the chairman, General Sir Gordon MacMillan, announced the Effort for Erskine fundraising scheme amid rekindled worries that Erskine would be unable to remain independent and would be absorbed into the NHS, thus losing its unique role. Fundraising was therefore specified as a part of the matron's duties. It was one Maureen took seriously. Visits to thank local groups or drum up support among more scattered branches of the Royal British Legion or veterans' associations became so frequent that Stuart remembers the younger children once offered to give all their pocket money to Erskine if that would allow their mother to spend an evening with them.

It was a necessary, sometimes onerous task but one which brought dividends. In 1978, donations from the public reached a high of £336,055. In later years, Stuart came to realise that not only was his mother very good at outlining Erskine's role but that both his parents enjoyed some of the social aspects of this part of the job.

Some of her predecessors had been sticklers for spit and polish beyond the requirements of hygiene; it was said that one would lay traps for cleaning staff by placing a dead fly out of immediate sight. Perhaps it was this image that made Maureen Lundie so determined to

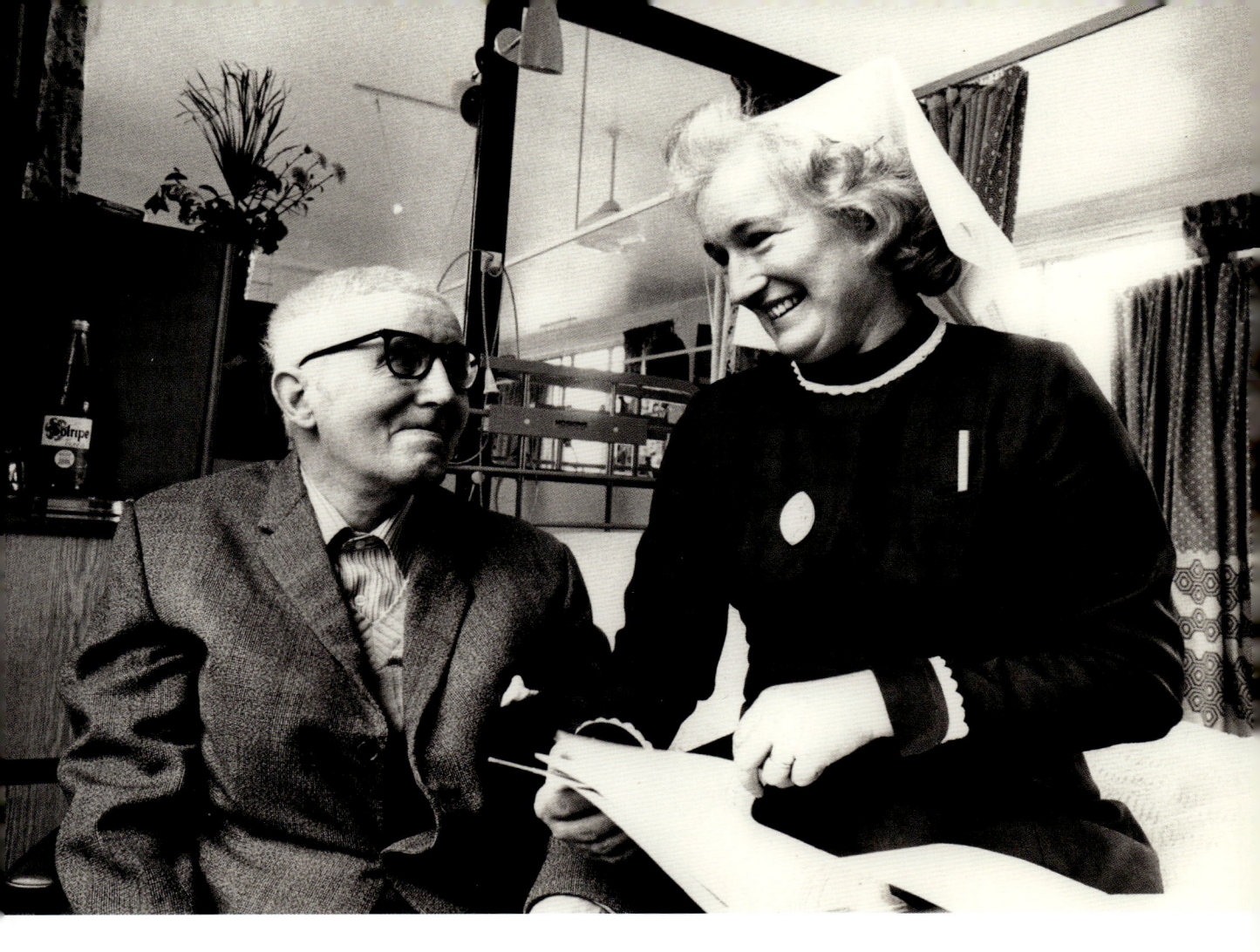

Matron Lundie gets a smile from a veteran of the Harvey Anderson Ward in the Erskine Hospital.

redefine the role of matron. She summed up her more practical approach in an interview after she was made OBE in 2000 for services to disabled former services personnel: "I went on ward rounds, although not to every ward and not at the same time. I really just walked round talking to people. The sisters had been trained in infection control and were responsible for hygiene in their wards and making sure the domestics did their job properly. I would intervene if I thought it necessary but I certainly didn't go about running my fingers along worktops looking for dust."

Nevertheless, she felt it was important to retain the title of matron. She had the chance to chance to change to director of nursing but said: "I wanted the patients at Erskine to realise that matrons are not all battleaxes." Stuart Lundie, however, experienced it from the staff's point of view. "My mother had a very distinctive step and when you heard her coming along the corridor you could tell what sort of mood she was in and there would be a rush to make sure everything was sparkling."

Despite the difficulties of the long Nightingale wards, one with 34 beds, both Stuart and Anne remember an exceptionally high standard of cleanliness with both nursing staff and domestics responsible for aspects of cleaning. "May Parks, the nursing officer, could have you cleaning the grout on the tiles with a toothbrush. She monitored cleanliness all the time and it worked," recalls Anne.

All six of the Lundie children worked in Erskine at various times, mostly in what was known as the students' job, a role which ranged from care assistant duties to cleaning.

Part of the learning process for these young people was that the camaraderie among residents and staff was often expressed in practical jokes. Stuart was the butt of one when told to feed a particular patient. The old soldier asked what was for pudding and when told "baked rice" ranted that he had spent years as a Japanese prisoner of war and never wanted to see another bowl of rice, greatly to the entertainment of the whole ward.

Anne is the only one of the six to follow in their mother's footsteps. She took a catering course when she left school but when between jobs worked as an auxiliary at Erskine. "I watched some fine people who were so good at their job and cared for everyone as an individual. They became my heroes," she says simply. Realising she wanted the satisfaction of caring for people, she applied to train as an enrolled nurse without telling her mother, who had always been careful never to put any pressure on her children to take up nursing. The secret was blown when her interview at the Western Infirmary coincided with a bus strike and a nurse offered a lift. To get time off, however, he had to explain to matron, who immediately summoned her husband to make sure Anne arrived on time. After qualifying, she returned to work at Erskine, to her mother's delight. Later Anne and two colleagues completed one of the first conversion courses to become registered nurses at the University of the West of Scotland financed by a loan from Erskine, where they continued to work. The hospital was so pleased with their excellent results that they were not required to repay the money. After that, a further 18 enrolled nurses took the course.

As Anne, who now manages the Day Hospital outpatients' clinics for Medicine for the Elderly at Drumchapel Hospital in Glasgow, points out, some of the measures that her mother implemented, such as active care plans and two-hourly checks, are now being brought in as required practice.

Although by this time there were few veterans who had lost limbs in the First World War, the hospital was still doing operations, including amputations, in the 1980s. Not until the 90s was it usual for patients to go out to other hospitals for operations or specialist treatment.

As even those who had served in the Second World War, reached old age, however, the focus was increasingly on care of the elderly. Maureen Lundie was one of the first people to campaign for women who had served in the forces to be eligible for medical and nursing care at Erskine on the same basis as the male veterans. In fact, there had never been a ban. The original limbless sailors and soldiers for whom the hospital was founded were, of course, all men and there had been no demand from women for many years. As a result, there was no suitable accommodation for women while Erskine was still run as a hospital with large wards and communal facilities.

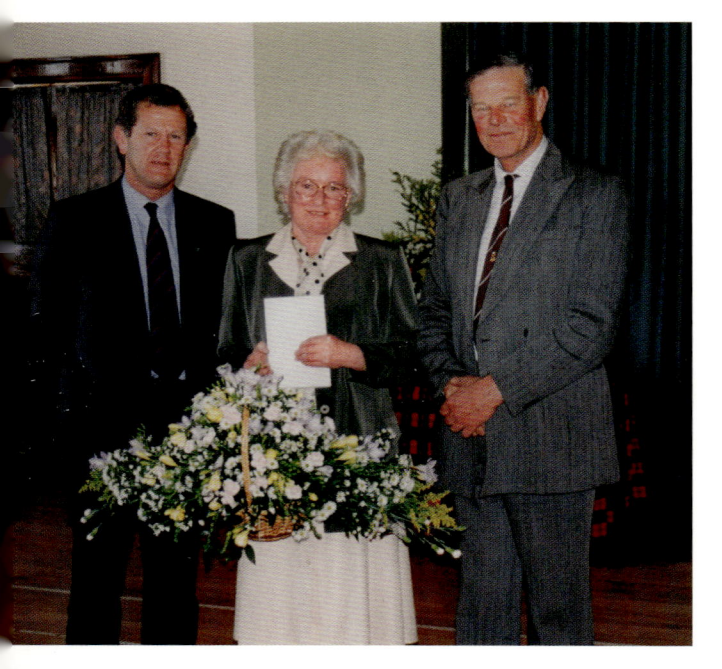

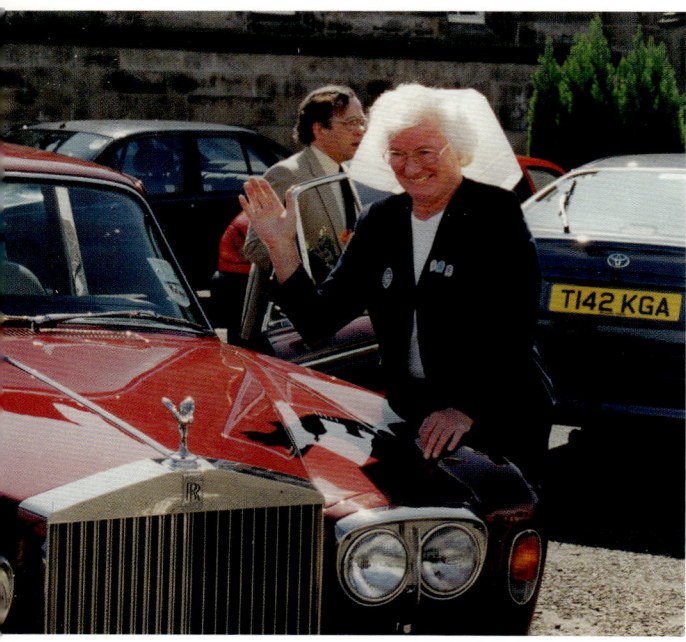

Top: After 22 years as matron, Maureen is presented with farewell gifts by Colonel Martin Gibson and Sir John MacMillan.

Above: She makes her final departure by red Rolls-Royce.

As the 469,000 women who had served in the Second World War reached old age, however, there was a need to extend care and in 1980 Elizabeth Watson, who had served with the Auxiliary Territorial Service (ATS) during the Second World War, became the first woman to be admitted as a permanent resident. Since then Erskine has welcomed a number of former ATS members as well as women from all three regular services. Today, nearly one-third of the residents are women and they include spouses of veterans as well as former servicewomen.

Stuart, as the youngest member of the Lundie family, remembers the wonderful freedom of a childhood with the run of the grounds but also the culture shock of being at eye-level with adults for the first time because so many of them were in wheelchairs. Living in "the creepiest house ever," however, was a mixed blessing. The fire escape route from one of the wards in the Mansion House was through the matron's quarters and the children became used to a confused patient occasionally wandering into their rooms.

Then there was the problem of everyone knowing exactly who he was and threatening to tell his mother whenever he was seen misbehaving. Unbeknown to Stuart, his summer activity of jumping in and out of the disused fishpond had been noted from an upstairs window. Summoned to his mother's office ("you always knew you were in trouble when she phoned and told you to go to the office"), his protests that this had only been a couple of times were useless in the face of a meticulous list of dates and times. The overwhelming memory for both Stuart and Anne, however, is of being part of the Erskine family, in which everyone on the estate, whatever their role, was a friend.

Their mother's maternal instinct extended not only to her six children but to the 300 patients and staff, encouraging everyone to make the most of their lives whether it was for patients to go on outings or staff to gain qualifications, with many gaining Scotvec qualifications (Scottish vocational certificates) on her watch.

It was just one more instance of the family atmosphere that residents, their families and staff all say is a distinguishing feature of Erskine. Although the military camaraderie has always been an important part of that, Maureen Lundie wanted to avoid the hospital being run on militaristic lines. "I always thought it was important that there was a lot of laughter because I wanted the residents to think of the place as their home." she said. Clearly far from being a battleaxe, she nevertheless fulfilled the traditional matron's role of knowing absolutely everything: "if there was a problem in the laundry room, you knew about it."

That commitment led to her staying on for a short while after retirement age to see the old hospital through its final stages before the patients were transferred to the new buildings. Her eventual retirement in 1999, brought heartfelt tributes to one of the hospital's best-loved matrons and a stylish send-off in a red Rolls-Royce.

Maureen Lundie was succeeded by Lorraine Ross who was responsible for the move of the patients from the Mansion House to the two new homes in Bishopton and Erskine in 2000 and later for the care of residents as they were admitted to the other homes as they were completed.

In 2011, the responsibility for nursing and care staff was taken on by Sue Robinson, whose title, director of care, reflects Erskine's shift of focus to elderly care, including dementia care as well as some residents with complex physical conditions. The increasingly rigorous standards laid down means a very detailed care plan must be in place for every resident and everything has to be recorded. Asked what would be the main difference between Maureen Lundie's time and her own she says: "Matrons who were in charge many years ago would be horrified by the amount of paperwork I have to do now."

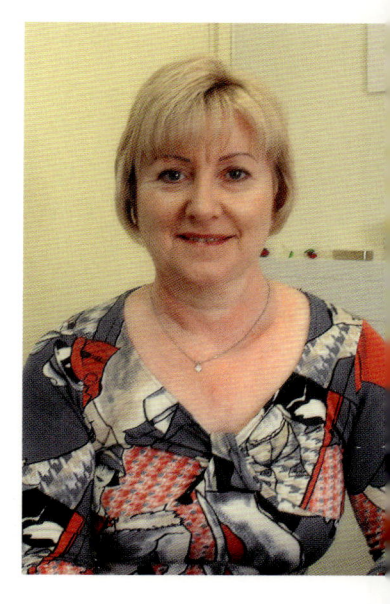

Lorraine Ross.

George Collins

"When I regained consciousness, I couldn't use my hands, talk or stand."

The remarkable story of George Collins is a reminder that our armed forces now risk life and limb in combat even where there has been no official declaration of war. The troop deployment to Northern Ireland that began as an emergency measure in August 1969 was to last 38 years, becoming the longest campaign in British military history and claiming the lives of 763 soldiers. It was a complicated conflict with no clear battle lines but it wrought 6116 wounded casualties, many as severely mutilated in body and as cruelly damaged in mind as those of the First and Second World Wars.

A Glasgow boy, George Collins had always wanted to be a soldier and joined the Argyll and Sutherland Highlanders at the first opportunity. Once in the regiment, he relished the opportunity to learn new skills including driving and radio operations and, full of enthusiasm, extended his contract to 22 years. He accumulated a variety of experiences in a short time from guarding the Queen at Balmoral to guarding Rudolf Hess in Spandau. When the Argylls were disbanded, he joined the Royal Highland Fusiliers and was posted with them to Northern Ireland for the first time in 1970.

After the success of the high-profile "Save the Argylls" campaign, he rejoined the regiment and was dispatched to Northern Ireland for a second tour. By a devastating quirk of fate, he was chosen, because of his signalling skills, from those volunteering to take the place of a colleague who was too ill to go on border patrol on the night of September 10, 1972. In the maze of country roads between the two parts of Ireland their armoured Saracen car was blown up by a 500lb landmine. The vehicle flew over a hedge and landed in a field. The radio on George's back lodged 50 feet up in a tree while he lay trapped beneath colleagues unable to move for an hour until a woman driving a Mini got stuck in the crater the bomb had left and shouted for help, alerting another patrol.

Three of his colleagues were killed. Amazingly, a further three, once freed, were relatively uninjured. George, however, had severe injuries, including paralysis of his right side and brain damage from lack of oxygen. When his wife Joy first saw him in hospital in Belfast: "His head was all bandaged up and he was like a balloon," she says. She knew the swollen cocooned figure was her handsome young soldier only because he had an eagle tattooed on his forearm. The couple were only recently married. They were engaged at 17 and George had accepted Joy's father's stipulation that they must wait until she was 20 before they married. He relented when George was due to be posted to Singapore. Joy was 19 and George 20, when they tied the knot, little imagining that within four years both their lives were changed for ever by that mine.

She hands over a leaflet with a photograph of her then fiancé as part of the Queen's Balmoral guard and leaves the room on the pretext of looking for another document. Like so many photographs of young men killed or wounded in action, the 19-year-old's good looks speak volumes of what might have been.

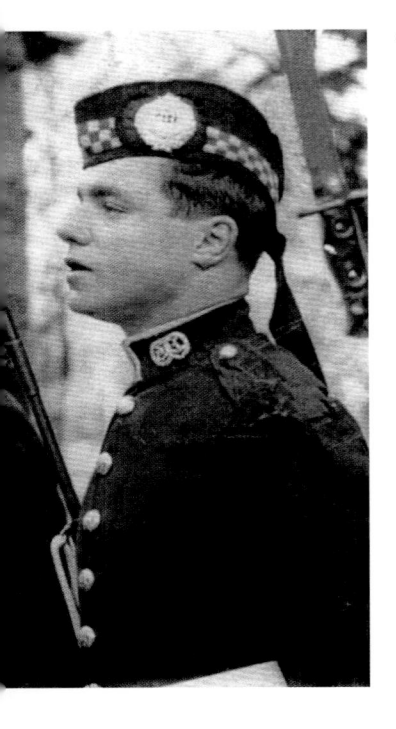

George Collins as a 19-year-old on royal guard duty at Balmoral.

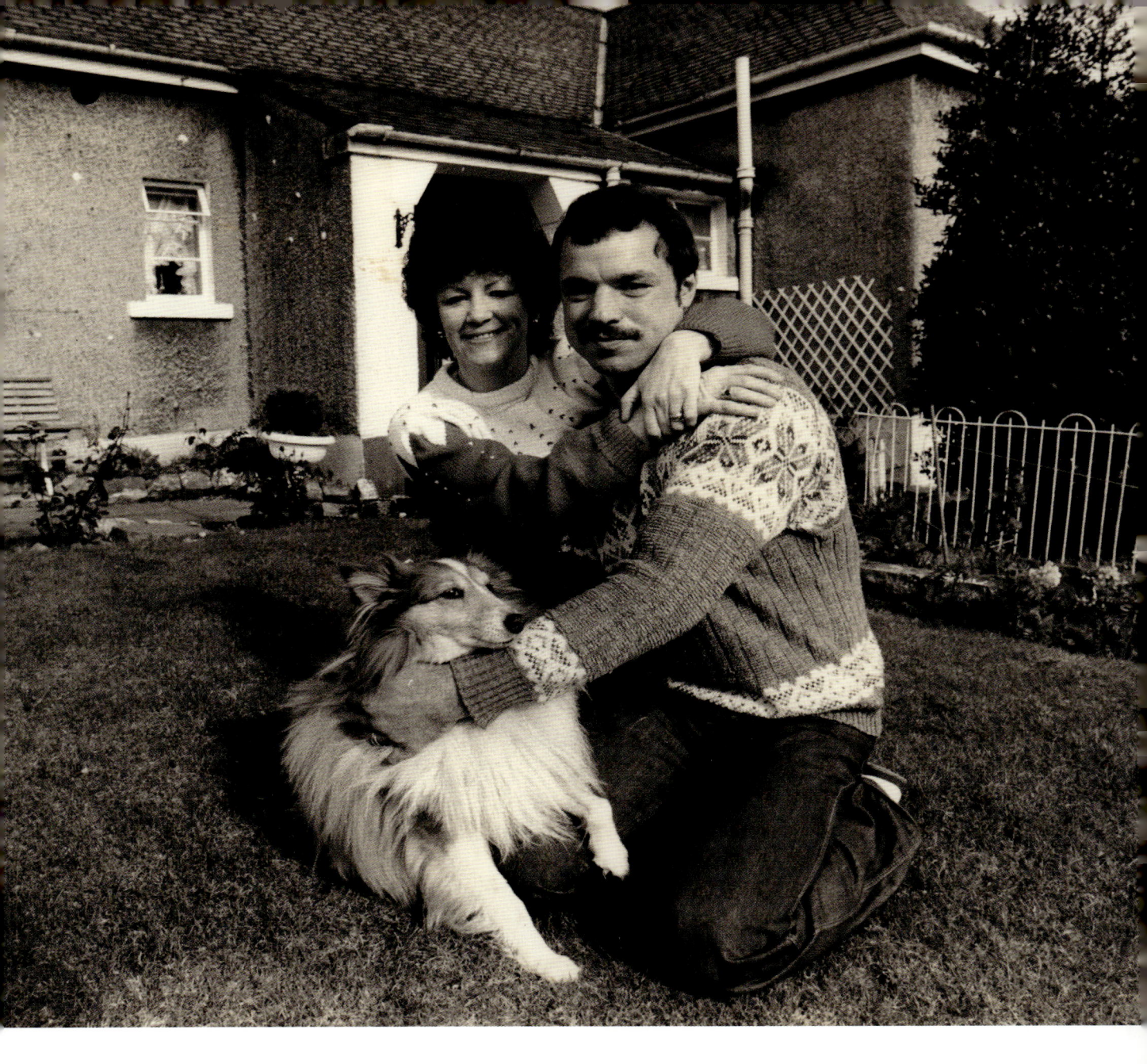

A house at Erskine enabled George and Joy to rebuild their life together

In his case, the reality was initial treatment in Belfast, followed by further operations in a military hospital in Woolwich and rehabilitation at RAF Chessington, now the specialist joint services rehabilitation centre Headley Court. In all, this took about a year and Joy was keen for him to return home. That prospect, however, posed severe practical difficulties. She had found a flat in Glasgow but it would not be able to accommodate her husband in his wheelchair. It was her father, an ambulanceman who knew of Erskine from taking patients there, who suggested George might be eligible for a place. More than 40 years later, the relief and gratitude still shine from her face as she explains that they were able to move into a cottage that was not only suitably adapted but detached so that she did not have to worry about neighbours being disturbed by George's nightmares.

He takes up the story explaining that, at the time, Erskine was still being run as a hospital with its own medical staff. Having physiotherapy on site enabled him to move on from his wheelchair to a walking frame, to two sticks, then one and eventually to walk

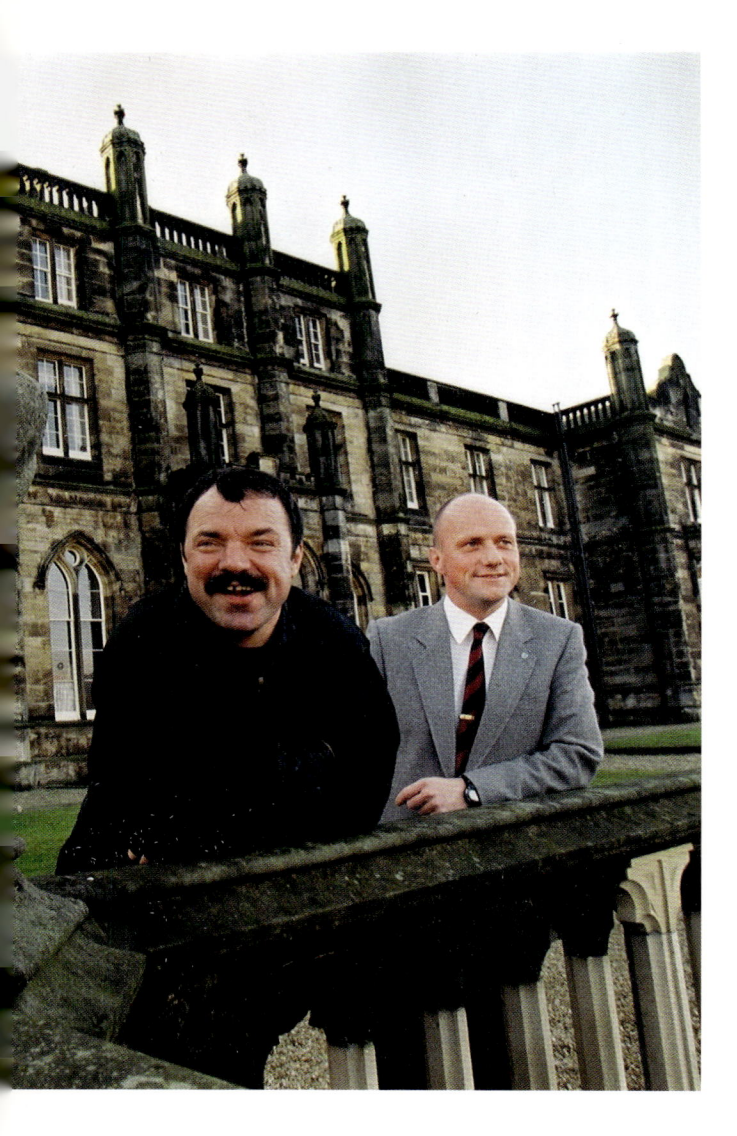

George (left) with fellow Erskine resident, Bill McDowall, outside the mansion house.

unaided, albeit with an awkward gait due to a twisted foot. When he complains that he can no longer run or swim, a cheerful grin contradicts the regretful shake of the head because the progress he's made as a result of dogged determination amounts to a heroic victory against adversity. He's done a variety of useful jobs over the years, ranging from making purses in occupational therapy to working as a print assistant and in the garden centre. It is no longer economic for Erskine, as a charity, to run these sheltered employment companies but George's growing skills are now put to use in Gardening Leave, a new charity which uses the physical exercise and sense of achievement in growing food as therapy for veterans recovering from injury or suffering from post-traumatic stress or disabling psychiatric conditions as a result of their experiences in conflict. The original veterans' garden centre has successfully been taken over by a commercial company but is a good neighbour, encouraging donations to Erskine in its shop. Gardening Leave is an example of the organic development of Erskine. Its Glasgow garden is on the Erskine site, facilitating interaction between the two service charities. George is the perfect go-between. Despite his limitations, he has retained the can-do attitude that made him such a good fit for Army life all those years ago: "I can show them how to plant. I can show them how to look after plants."

At a time when large care facilities, whether for the frail elderly, physically disabled people or those with psychiatric illnesses, are being replaced with care at home, it is worth noting that George found inspiration and encouragement from being in a community with others facing similar problems. His progress was not a seamless process. There were real difficulties and, in the early years, the inevitable frustration of a young man who had expected to lead an active and adventurous life finding himself dependent on others and not always able to express himself completely and coherently.

Joy explains: "Our next-door neighbour when we moved in had no legs. Yet he had the most beautiful garden. He used to take off his artificial legs and move about on what we called a boogie board. It helped George to move from thinking about the negatives all the time to seeing the positives." He surprised himself by taking up bowls. After seeing others playing in spite of missing limbs, he took on the challenge by adapting the technique of a double amputee: getting down on his knees and clutching the wood between his numb fists. It was a breakthrough moment in understanding that not only must he relearn basic skills like walking and talking but that it was also important to learn new ones.

Recently, for the first time in 40 years, George came face-to-face with the soldier whose place he took that fateful night. Of course it was emotional but it was also a surprisingly joyful occasion. George has a constant struggle with his memory and couldn't recognise the man. It was clear that the situation had weighed heavily on his conscience over the decades. "He came in and said: You must hate me," recalled Joy. Having been tested as severely as her husband over the years, her answer was simple, blunt and practical. "I don't hate anybody.

I detest the people who planted that mine but they later blew themselves up with their own explosives. I certainly don't hate Irish people. Like most people in the west of Scotland, some of my ancestors came from Ireland and how can you hate a whole country?"

She adds: "A lot of George's unit had wanted to visit but they were frightened of what they were going to see." That is understandable among young men facing danger as part of their working lives. The toll of conflict is difficult to live with and forces all service personnel to question what they are doing. The reality of George's useful life in defiance of his extensive injuries was a surprise and delight for his former colleagues, not least because he and Joy have built a happy family life at Erskine. Despite being told they would not be able to have children, they have successfully raised two daughters, now both working (one as a nurse specialising in neurological injuries). Both parents say they could not have done this without the security of the Erskine community around them. "There was no way George could have made it, if he'd just gone back to Civvy Street. He found noise really difficult…" Joy's explanation tails off. Other problems remain unspoken but the bustle and impatience of modern life is more likely to exacerbate than alleviate the complex needs of wounded service personnel.

Joy now feels it is important to support others in the way they were encouraged when they first arrived. She runs social activities and is long-practised at persuading residents who tend to be more reclusive than is healthy to join others for outings or go to the ceilidhs her group organises. While she cheerfully says she doesn't take "no" for an answer, her own experience makes her highly sensitive to the needs of others. "There are some people who just don't want to go out after dark. I understand that. They like security, so I work my way round that so they can come out for lunch or we arrange to go the pictures in the afternoon."

Along with fundraising, this is Joy's way of repaying Erskine for all they've done: "They gave us a house and they gave George a job and they raised our two girls. The great thing about Erskine is they don't treat people like invalids, they treat them like men." Over the years, the couple have often been introduced to visiting royalty. George and Joy were particularly delighted to be able to show the Prince of Wales round their home. Coincidentally, they were also invited to a garden party at Buckingham Palace that summer. This is the cue for one of George's favourite tales: When Prince Charles told George "Your face is familiar," he received the unexpected reply: "Well, you came to see us in our house a few weeks ago, so we thought we would come and see you in yours." Joy hastily says: "I was mortified" but the happy smile gives the game away. She was – and is – proud of her husband. Those flashes of humour and cheeky personality are not just proof of rehabilitation but are her reward for long years of courage and loyalty.

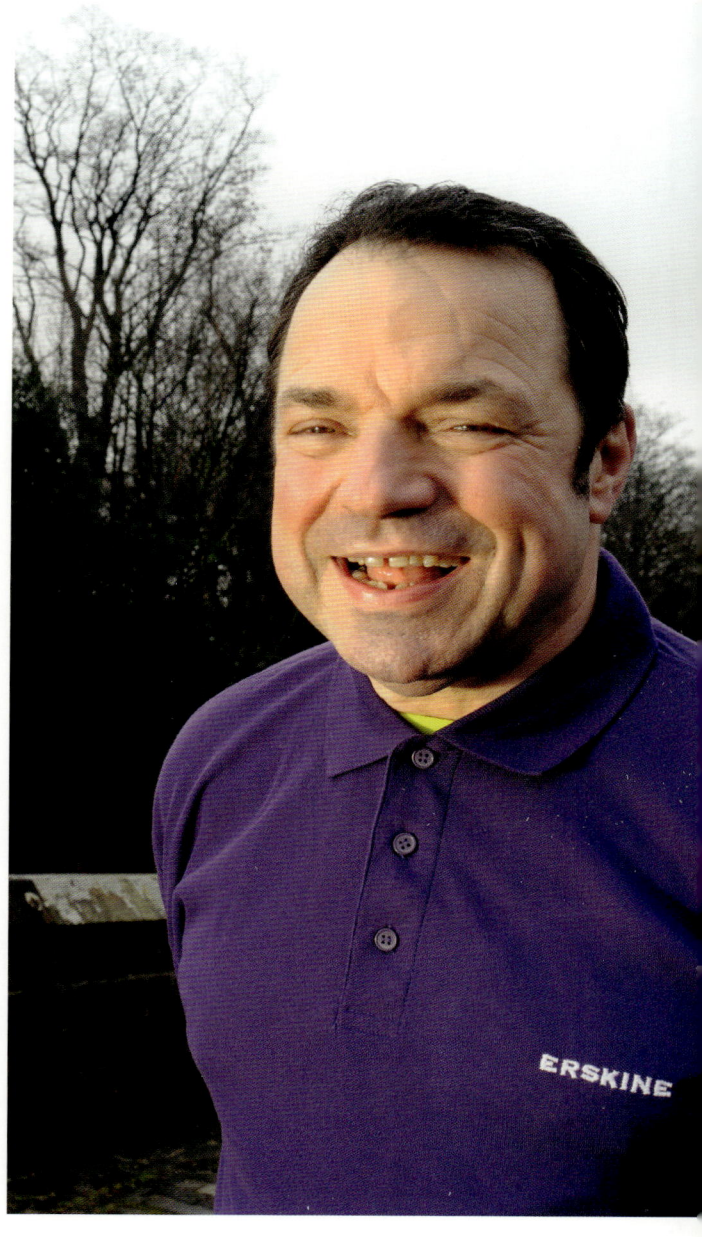

George is delighted to pass on his gardening knowledge to other injured veterans.

Dr Thomas McFadyen

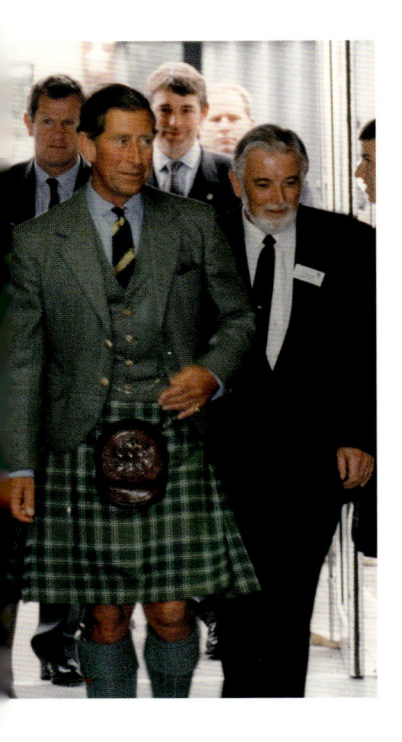

"The longest patient I had died after he'd been here 47 years. He had no one else; we were his family. And that's the way we treated the patients, as if they were part of our family. Erskine becomes a way of life."

Dr Tom McFadyen escorts Prince Charles on a visit to the hospital.

In Mar Hall, the luxurious hotel on the banks of the Clyde, Dr Tom McFadyen navigates his way confidently through the lavishly appointed rooms, describing the history of each in turn.

It is an inspiring story of the pragmatic response to a crisis that threatened to overwhelm the medical facilities available in Scotland in 1916. Having spent 25 years as the chief medical officer in this building in its former life as a hospital and specialist care home for ex-servicemen, he sees rows of beds where today there is a comfortable tearoom. As the testimony of war veterans, particularly amputees, nursed in the Nightingale wards of what was then Erskine Hospital makes clear, however, there has long been a plentiful supply of tea and solicitude and a century of five-star service in this long gallery with its breathtaking river views. "You felt the atmosphere of history as soon as you walked in," he says but it is soon evident that his most powerful recollection is the sense of community. "If you met someone in the corridor you spoke to them. If you passed a patient you always said hello. I knew every patient by their first name." From the beginning, the unique mission of the charity to treat the "limbless sailors and soldiers" of the First World War, the extraordinary level of public support and the parkland setting of the former mansion house gave it a very different atmosphere from conventional hospitals.

Dr McFadyen first became involved with Erskine while working at the Royal Alexandra Hospital in Paisley, where he was increasingly interested in geriatric medicine and switched from his original speciality of dermatology. Regular visits to Erskine became part of his workload when the chief medical officer at the hospital became ill. When the post became vacant, he was appointed, the first non-military holder of the post. He relished the wide range of cases he had to deal with and, because they could offer excellent post-operative care, Erskine was still carrying out surgical operations, sometimes major ones, using visiting surgeons.

The First World War veterans who had remained at Erskine because they were too incapacitated to return to the community he recalls as great characters. One, nicknamed Jutland because he had been torpedoed at the Battle of Jutland, told Prince Charles that he had been on the ship commanded by his uncle, Lord Mountbatten. Erskine's royal patron questioned some detail of the old sailor's account and vowed to check with his uncle. On his next visit, the prince sought out Jutland to admit his version had been confirmed.

As the remaining original patients reached old age and even those who had fought in the Second World War became pensioners, Dr McFadyen worked with Maureen Lundie, the matron at the time, to improve the facilities and tailor medical services to meet patients' individual needs which were identified during the regular ward rounds they instituted.

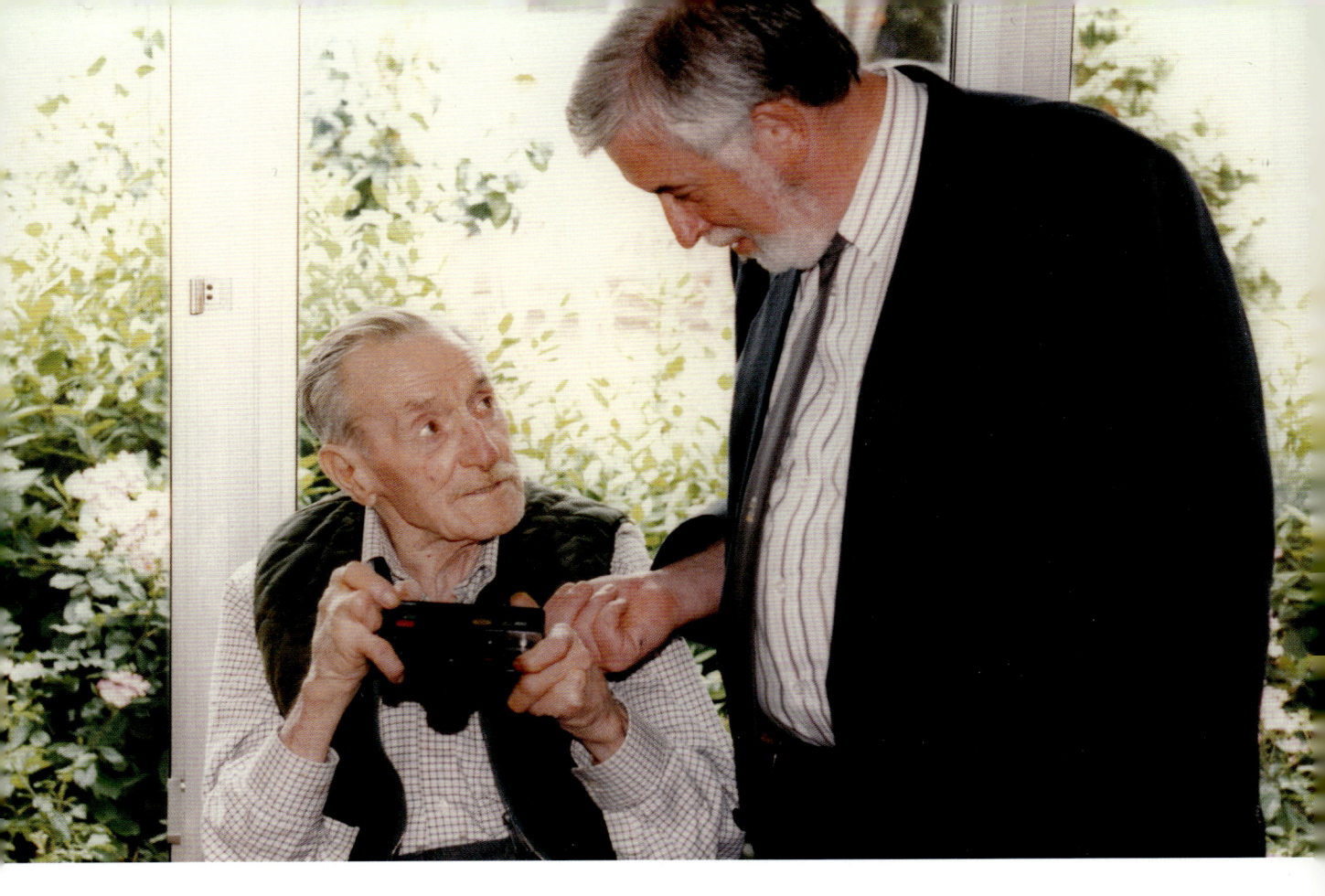

Perhaps more significant in the long term was the creation of Erskine's own physiotherapy department. To this day, Erskine residents have access to physiotherapy without having to rely on the severely-stretched NHS services. The expertise gained in working with disabled veterans is also available to residents whose mobility has been affected by age-related conditions and physiotherapy on site is one of the major advantages of Erskine compared with other care homes

"Although some of them were over 100, I never thought of them as old people. To me, they were always my patients, they were all treated the same, whether they were 28 or 100." His emphasis on improving the quality of life, not just medical care, extended his remit beyond that of doctor to the role of organiser and fundraiser for additional facilities.
A project to which he devoted considerable time was the holiday home in Dunoon which provided a welcome change of scenery for those unable to travel or without family to visit. This was especially beneficial for long-term patients and one more example of how Erskine became not just a treatment centre for veterans but a community in which every patient felt welcome.

From the medical practitioner's point of view, this caring atmosphere made it an exceptionally rewarding place in which to live and work. "Erskine becomes a way of life. It was like a family. You didn't know what the day was going to bring when you arrived down at the hospital but that's what made it exciting. The longest patient I had died after he'd been there 47 years. He had no one else; we were his family. And that's the way we treated the patients, as if they were part of our family." They reciprocated. When his parents came to visit at his house on the estate, they would go to the canteen to buy their papers and

Discussions with the Doc were not confined to medical matters. Dr McFadyen examines a camera with a veteran from the Lauder Thomson Ward in The Erskine Hospital.

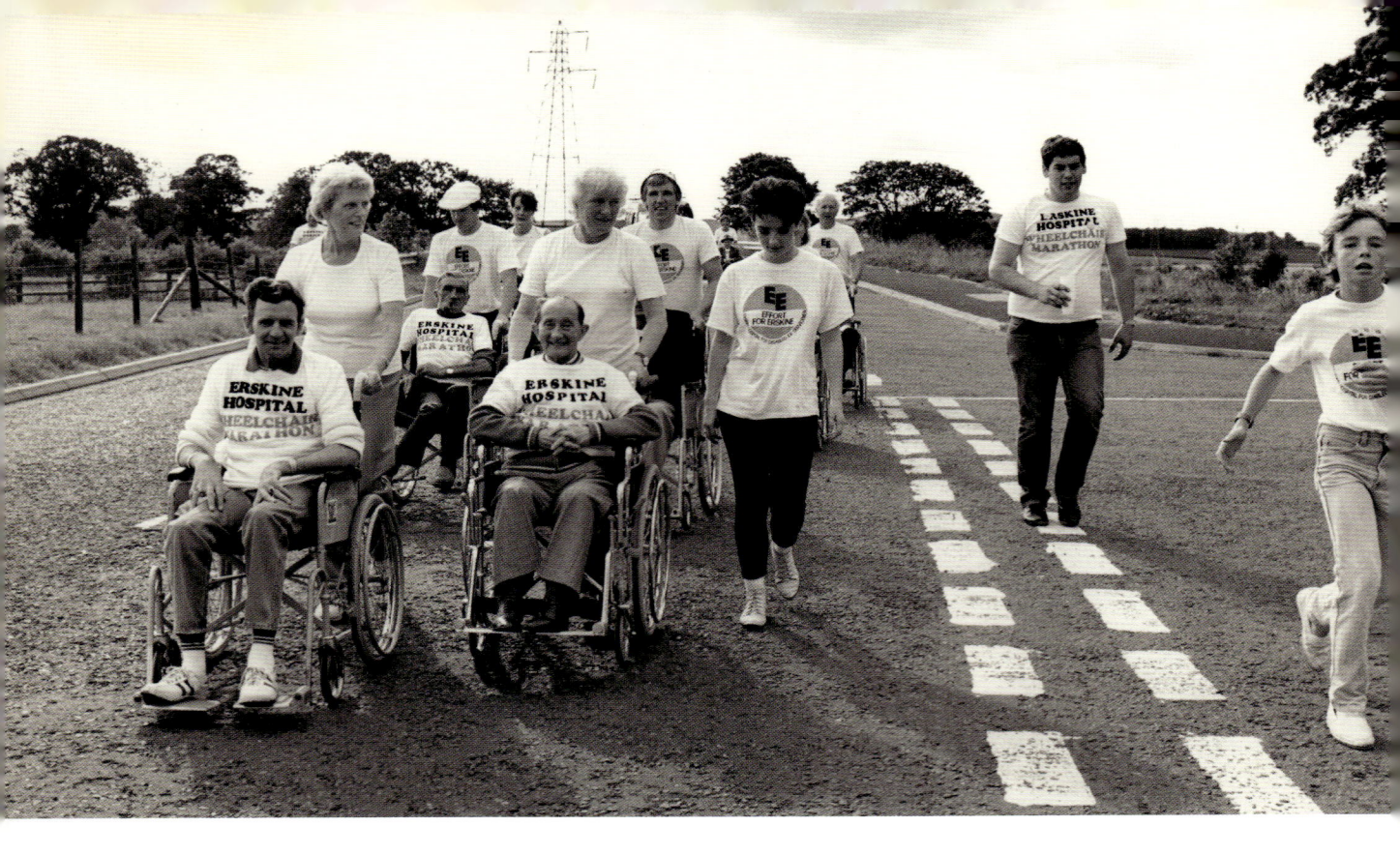

The wheelchair marathon was a fundraising success and a highlight of the year for staff and residents.

spend all morning chatting to the residents. Soon they were giving him small presents, such as tomatoes they had grown, to pass on to his mother.

He recalls the camaraderie the physical conditions engendered as a positive element of care. "Because the veterans were already used to living in close-quarters from their time in the army, they enjoyed the open wards of the mansion house. In those days, there was a camaraderie among the patients and staff." That can be true in any hospital ward where a robust cheeriness helps alleviate unavoidable indignities but the spirit of Erskine which pervaded the grand old building amounted to a deeper companionship, albeit in the day-to-day ordinariness of bedside chats, tea breaks accompanied by horoscope predictions or (a reminder of a different age) a smoke.

This culture of comradeship was not the only difference from other hospitals. Erskine's distinct identity was cultivated outwith the National Health Service and the demands of hierarchical management. As a charity governed by trustees, the senior staff had considerable freedom. In Tom McFadyen's words, which suggest he shared the direct approach of his great predecessor Sir William Macewen: "We were able to run the place the way it needed to be run, not the way some bureaucrat thought it should be run. Matron Lundie and I instilled a get-things-done attitude in the medical and nursing staff."

Such independence, however, meant there was no central funding and the medical department had to raise the money to provide the high level of care that was their goal. Thus a Saturday morning could find the chief medical officer abseiling down the walls of Stirling Castle in exchange for £800. Tom retains particularly fond memories of the annual wheelchair marathon, despite it usually taking place in blistering heat or drenching rain. Whatever the weather, the format was invariable. Staff would line up ten to 15 patients in wheelchairs outside the mansion house. Encouraged by the cheers of the remaining staff and patients, they set off on the 20-mile round trip to Paisley. "We would go by the back road to Bishopton, round by the airport to the centre of Paisley and stop in the council offices car park. I drove back to Erskine to pick up the lovely hot soup and sandwiches the kitchen staff made for us and we would have a picnic in the car park before going down the main street, through Renfrew and past the airport. Crowds on the roadside always filled the donation buckets. I would be directing the traffic and I never once had a complaint from a motorist about being held up. Instead, because people could see the wheelchair bus covered in posters, they would often roll down their windows and stuff a £10 note into my hands. As well as raising a lot of money, it was great fun. They were all clapped back in when they got to Erskine, the kitchen made us fish and chips and the bottles of champagne were opened."

Dr McFadyen acknowledges the generosity of the neighbouring community has been vital to Erskine's success. His dedication was an equally crucial factor over the quarter century when, inevitably, given the demands of the job, the hospital became a major part of his life. "I rarely had time for interests outside the hospital, I was on call 24 hours a day," he says. In the days before mobile phones, he could be summoned by pager if away from Erskine.

The most dramatic instance of this was during a visit to the opera in Glasgow. "It was a performance of Tosca. The audience was holding its breath in anticipation as it reached its denouement. And just as Tosca was about to fling herself over the parapet, my pager went off. I had to crawl out in great embarrassment and find a phone."

One of the emergencies he handled as CMO was a salmonella outbreak at the hospital, a potentially disastrous situation if the infection was not contained. After closing wards, he was still carrying out administrative tasks at 2am. "That's the kind of thing you had to do because there was nobody else and that was that."

Over the years, the Doc, as the residents liked to call him ("Son" was another favourite) says there was not much you didn't see in terms of illness. Yet however challenging particular conditions might be or whatever the satisfaction in averting a full-scale crisis from an outbreak of infection, this dedicated medic has the simplest of answers to the question of what was the most rewarding aspect of his work. Without hesitation, he says: "Getting a smile from the patients."

One long-time colleague recalled a piece of advice Dr McFadyen gave her when she started work at Erskine: "Always give them a smile because it may be the last one they'll ever see." She took this to heart and would always wish the patients farewell with a big smile. His words have resonated poignantly for her since the day she went on duty to find an apparently healthy patient had died in the night and it's a motto that remains with staff to this day.

Despite retiring over a decade ago, Tom can't pass through the modern Erskine without recognising an old face and receiving many waves from friends and former colleagues. "I never missed the work but always missed the patients. I used to come down here and see people anyway. I'd come and walk down the corridor, and see the patients I knew, and they'd say: 'Aw, I wish you were back, Doc' and the staff would say: 'Aw, I wish you were here, it's not the same without you' and that always meant something to me, hoping that I had made a mark on them all."

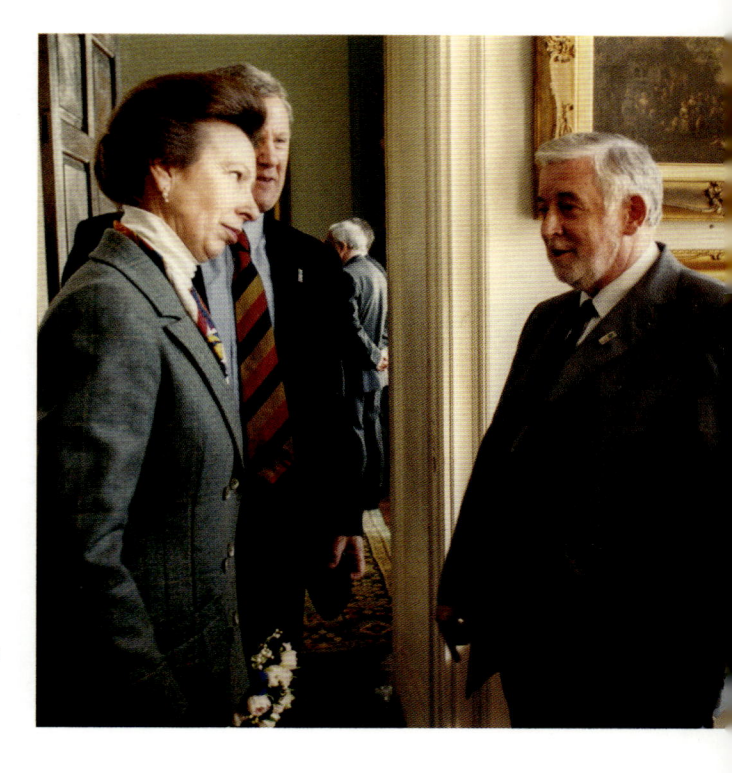

On royal duty, Dr McFadyen outlines Erskine's unique qualities to Princess Anne.

Isobel Kirkwood

"All my friends have passed on and my family live in Manchester, so Erskine is my life now."

Erskine could not exist without its army of volunteers who raise funds and provide many of the services that make it so special. Step forward Isobel Kirkwood.

Though she is only three years younger than Erskine itself, Isobel will do anything to support her favourite good cause. Well, almost anything. Recently she drew the line at dangling over the River Clyde from a giant crane on the basis that she does not own a pair of trousers and had no desire to flash her underwear at the crowd below!

It is commonplace to describe cogent active nonagenarians as "spry" or "game" but such clichés don't seem to fit this formidable ex-head teacher who can still hold a class of youngsters spellbound for 90 minutes with her accounts of the Blitz and being courted by a dashing Scottish Spitfire pilot; and who raises thousands of pounds a year for Erskine, ably abetted by her King Charles spaniel and his begging bowl; and who thinks nothing of spending hours stuffing envelopes and helping out several days each week in the Erskine fundraising office. As one young Erskine employee told her: "We don't think of you as old at all."

Gerontologists now believe that helping others is the single best way for the over-70s to prolong active meaningful life. Isobel agrees: "All my friends have passed on and my family live in Manchester, so Erskine is my life now."

She was the second of three sisters, born in London of Aberdonian parents. Their father worked for the GPO. Apart from a bout of scarlet fever at age five, she remembers a happy childhood of ballet and piano lessons, lots of reading and simple pleasures like homemade lemonade.

As a teenager in the 1930s she was uninterested in politics but seeing the film of Noel Coward's Cavalcade, with its scenes of London in WW1, left her with a lasting fear of war and newsreels of Nazi soldiers goose-stepping through Berlin haunted her.

By 1938 she was training to be a teacher. "War was coming. I remember walking round the grounds of the college with my history tutor and sharing my fears. She said I'd be too busy with the children to be scared and would soon adapt."

She was right. Isobel embarked on her first job, at Southall in Middlesex, in August 1940 at the height of the Battle of Britain. "So there I was in an air raid shelter in the playground with 52 five-year olds and the sound of Spitfires taking off from RAF Northolt nearby. Air raids became part of normal life. The children sat on long benches and spent the days chanting nursery rhymes and learning letters and numbers, with nothing more than a blackboard and chalk. But they didn't know any different. Anyway, they could all read by the end of the school year."

On September 7 1940, she was watching Sir Henry Wood conduct the London Symphony Orchestra at the Queen's Hall, when there was an announcement: "London is burning." She emerged to an orange sky and the crump of bombs falling on the docks.

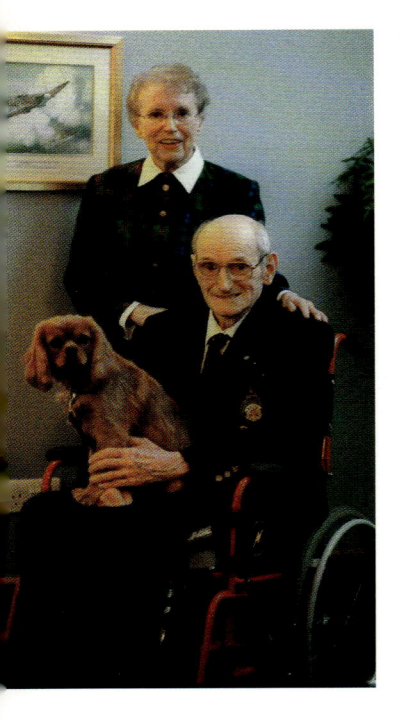

Isobel with Robert and Harry at Erskine.

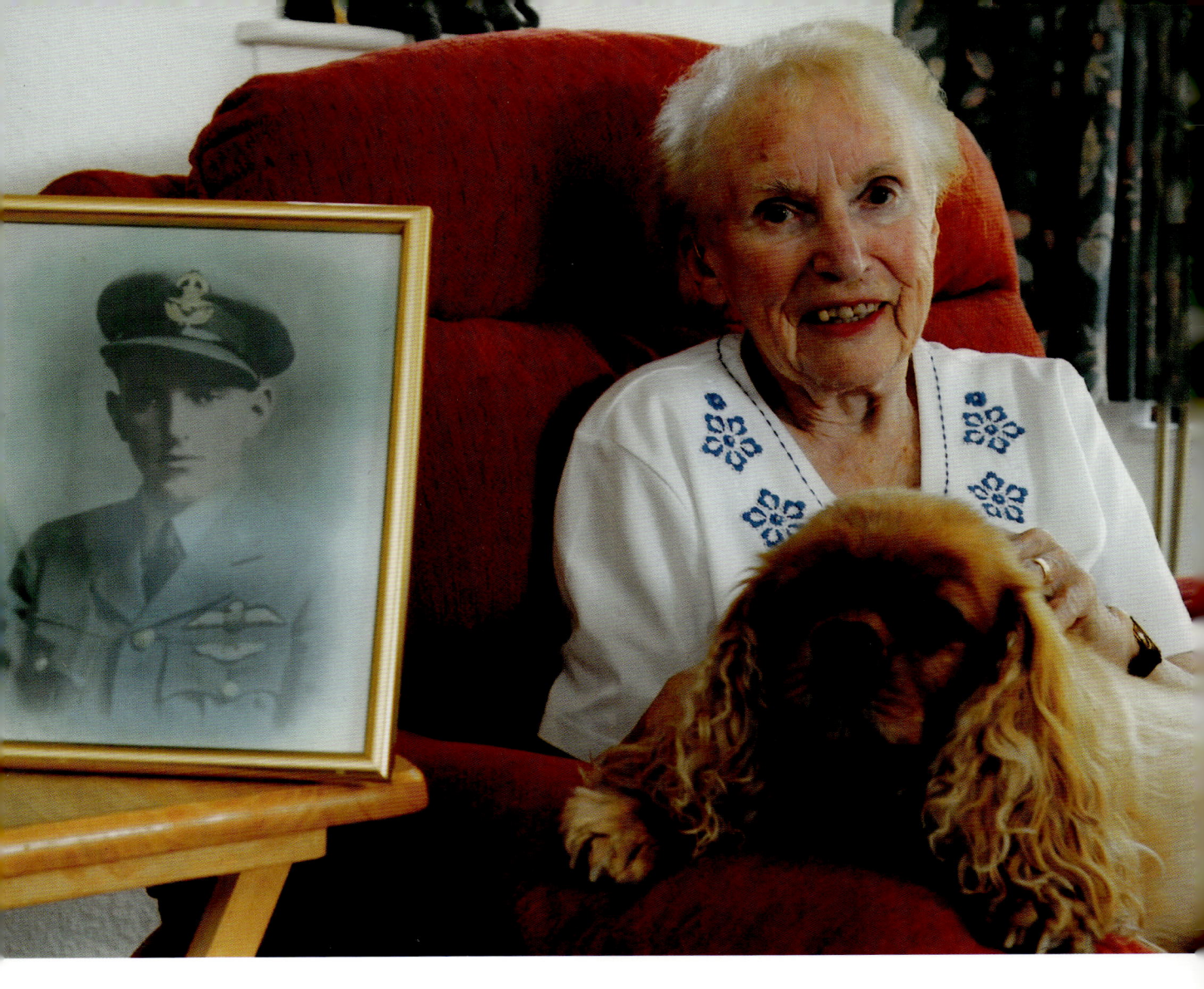

A chance invitation from her old college to spend a holiday in the residence to which it had been evacuated in South Devon, would change her life forever. "It was a joy to find the area inundated with 'boys in blue' (RAF trainees)," she confides. At a dance, she met Robert Kirkwood, a baker's son from Irvine, who had joined the RAF at 18. ("You must admit, he's smashing," she says, flaunting his photo in uniform.)

Subsequent evenings wandering along the local clifftops at dusk were less romantic than they sound. "He was trying to study aircraft recognition and I left for London not knowing if I'd ever see him again." A great dancer, Robert proved a hopeless letter writer. But, though hotly pursued by a Washington Post war correspondent for the next two years, Isobel couldn't forget Robert. ("The American may have been a great writer but he was a terrible dancer!")

Such had been the attrition rate among pilots during the Battle of Britain that aircrews were sent all over the place for training. Robert was soon wearing the solid silver wings of the American Air Corps. He and Isobel met again briefly in late 1942 before he sailed from the Clyde to join 111 Squadron in Tunis. She wouldn't see him again until October 1944.

Did she fear for his life? No, ignorance was bliss, it seems: "It wasn't like WW1 when newspapers were full of casualty lists. Now news was controlled. To us, Dunkirk was brave

Isobel with her cherished photograph of Robert in his RAF uniform and Rusty her King Charles spaniel.

Isobel Kirkwood 69

little boats, not bodies on beaches. Everyone was separated from those they loved and you knew anything could happen. You only found out about terrible things later. Robert saw a ship torpedoed going through the Straits of Gibraltar. He saw Wrens drowning while the rest of the convoy went on. It had to."

Was she ever frightened for herself? There were near misses. One day the children came to school to find their air raid shelter reduced to rubble. Her local (mercifully empty) cinema was flattened. "Somehow you always expected the bomb to fall on someone else, someone you didn't know." But on May 11 1943 there was a direct hit on the ATS (Auxiliary Territorial Service) hostel next to the Imperial Hotel in Great Yarmouth. It killed her best friend Enid and 25 other young women. That was one of the blackest days of Isobel's war.

In June 1944 the first of the Doodlebugs (V1 drones) blew out all the windows in her parents' home. "But I think the most frightening moment had been after Dunkirk when a Government leaflet came through the door, telling us what to do if the Germans invaded. My blood ran cold and I realised what we were up against."

After chasing the Germans across North Africa, Robert and his fellow Spitfire pilots in 111 Squadron were in Sicily preparing to protect the bombers as the Allies retook Italy. "The distance from Sicily to Salerno gave them only half an hour over the target. Their plans were seemingly leaked because it took them ten days flying back and forth to establish the beachhead. By that time all the surviving pilots had dysentery and piles!" Then Robert contracted malaria in Egypt. "By the time he was flown home in September 1944, he weighed barely six stone. "I hardly recognised him," says Isobel. A kind head teacher gave her unofficial leave and the couple went to Scotland. "I came back wearing an engagement ring."

Isobel and Robert married in London in March 1945 as Monty crossed the Rhine. ("Every stitch was borrowed except my knickers.") They celebrated with the first ice cream Isobel had tasted since 1939. Their son Roger was born on Boxing Day, nine months and two days later.

The killing had stopped but there was still rationing and hardship. In fact, for the Kirkwood family, life was about to take a terrible turn. Having settled in Robert's home town of Irvine, Isobel felt isolated and friendless. Classed as a Scottish girl in England, in Scotland she was labelled as English and given the cold shoulder, a common problem for Anglo-Scots.

Then came what seemed like a worse bombshell than anything unleashed by Hitler. Robert was diagnosed with what we now know as multiple sclerosis. His life expectancy was put at ten years maximum.

Robert and Isobel made several major decisions. Isobel would go back to teaching. They would keep Robert's condition a secret from everyone, even their own son. And they would have no more children. Despite some problems getting her English qualifications accepted, she went on to spend 11 happy years working in Mosspark, before moves to several other primaries and ultimately a head teacher's job in King's Park, where she became a great favourite with parents, children and staff.

Roger got into Allan Glen's School and went on to graduate Bachelor of Architecture at Strathclyde University ("the proudest day of our lives since bringing him home as a new-born baby").

Meanwhile Robert's symptoms had seemingly miraculously disappeared and he was able to resume his career as a successful salesman of bakery equipment. His condition finally recurred in 1982 and this time there was no escape. "I took early retirement after 38 years in teaching so that I could drive him around until he retired," says Isobel. Soon Robert could no longer write and began falling, each time precipitating a call from Isobel to the police.

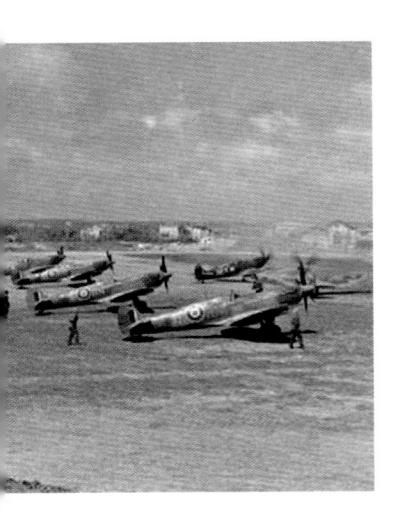

The 111 and 72 Squadron Spitfires in Italy.

"They would pick him up and were always charming but I knew we couldn't go on like this. Also, Robert's short-term memory was going."

The family GP suggested Erskine and Robert began by going there for respite care while Isobel grabbed the occasional holiday. Finally, in 1995 he left their immaculate bungalow in Newton Mearns for the last time and moved into Erskine permanently.

"The first year was hard. When I said I was going home, he'd say he would get his coat and come with me. I would drive home alone with tears welling. But it was like taking your child to school for the first time. I knew he was fine as soon as I'd gone. Soon he was calling all the nurses "honeybun" and all the male staff "curly", even if they were bald."

In the year 2000 when Erskine moved from Erskine House into a brand new purpose-built home with individual rooms, the Kirkwoods were introduced to Prince Charles, who asked Robert if he had ever been shot at. He nodded, adding "the shrapnel came through the floor of the plane and into my bum. There followed the best ten minutes of aerobatics you've ever seen!" Cue royal laughter.

Robert took to his new home. As Isobel says: "Everyone had a name on the door. That was their address. There were staff paid to create a social life for them and an events programme every day but nobody told them what to do and where to go. You'd never go and find a semi-circle of people waiting for their next meal. Everything has been thought out for the wellbeing of the residents. Erskine gives residents their lives back and gives them hope."

Since Robert's death in 2003 Erskine has given Isobel a new career. Ably abetted by Rusty, her King Charles spaniel, she raised more than £3000 for Erskine during Remembrance Week 2014, though even that pales beside more than £20,000 brought in by Rusty's predecessor, the much-lamented Harry.

Isobel continues to wow audiences with her wartime memories and to sing the praises of her favourite charity. Now that she no longer drives, staff from the Erskine fundraising office chauffeur her to these speaking engagements. "My toy boys" as she calls them and they love it.

As Erskine now welcomes the spouses of former service personnel, Isobel can look forward to coming there to live if the day ever arrives when she can no longer look after herself.

"My boys at Erskine think this is a great idea. They say they will come along after breakfast, dump me in a wheelchair and trundle me along to the office to start my day's work."

Her long dedication to Erskine was marked with the award of the British Empire Medal for services to veterans in Scotland in the New Year's Honours of 2016.

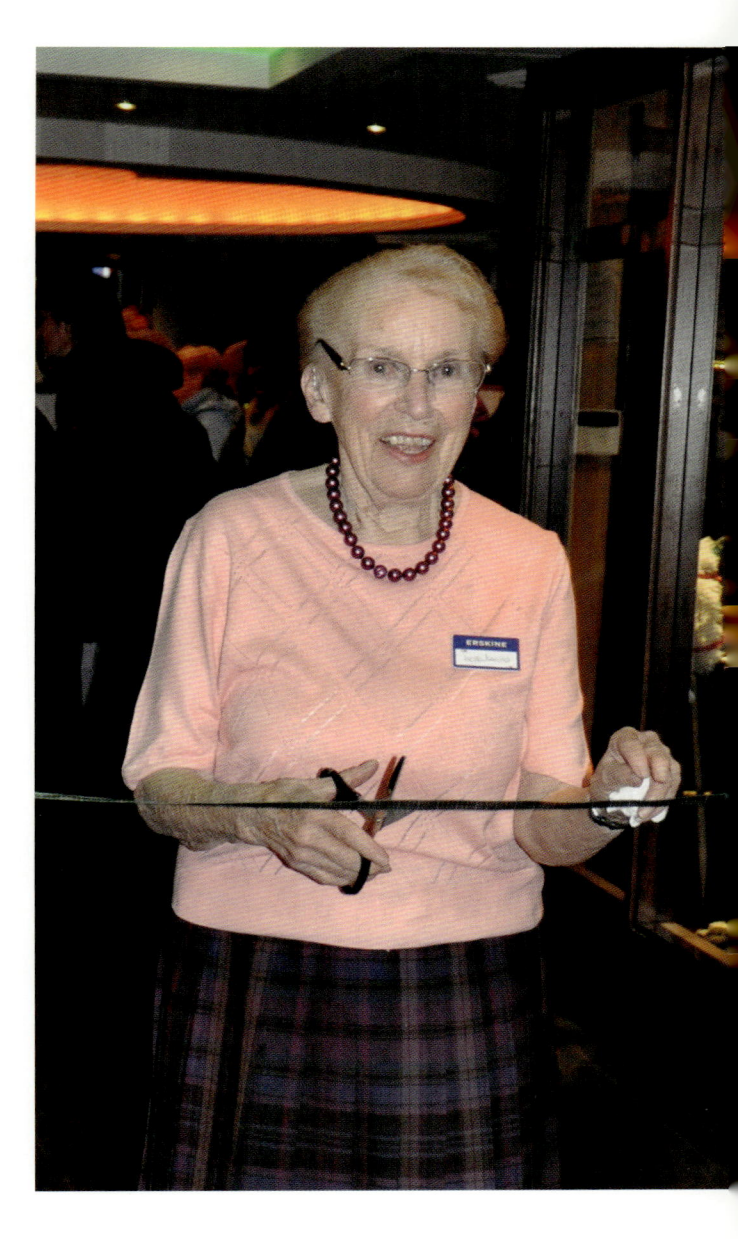

Cutting the ribbon to open the Erskine Christmas Cracker event in 2012.

Colonel Bobby Steele

"It was very much early 20th century as opposed to late 20th century. Things really had to change. Moving the hospital up the road was something I've always been proud of on behalf of the staff who embodied that old 'will-do' attitude: it had to be done, so they did it."

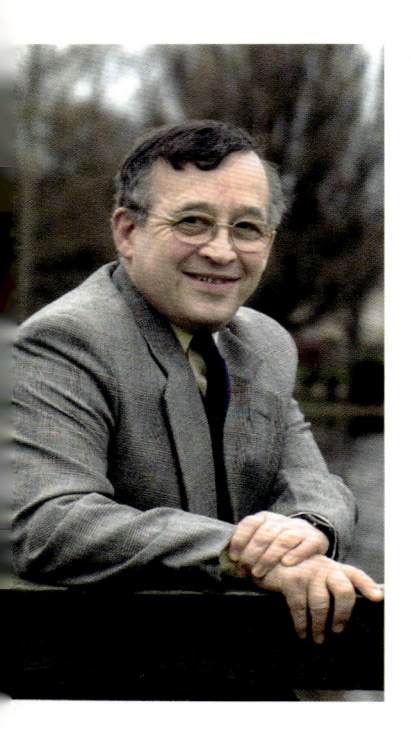

Colonel Bobby Steele, assistant commandant for 16 years, with "never a dull moment."

With a lifelong connection to the armed forces, Colonel Bobby Steele, says he is "quite well dug-in" to the veterans' community. That is an understatement. As assistant commandant at Erskine, from 1988 to 20004, he was a well-known figure to service charities.

His military career began at the age of 17 when he and his twin brother, David, trained at the Royal Military Academy Sandhurst. "We were of that post-war generation which all knew some sort of soldier and tales of derring-do abounded," he explains. His ambition to join the Cameronians was thwarted when the regiment was disbanded and he joined the Royal Corps of Transport, later transferring to the Argyll and Sutherland Highlanders.

His service included a tour of duty in Aden, which coincided with the Six-Day War in Israel in 1967. That had serious repercussions in Aden, where relations between the Arabs and British were strained by the suspicion that Britain as well as the US had aided Israel. Twenty-two British soldiers were killed in one day including eight members of Bobby Steele's squad of the Royal Corps of Transport. One was the second lieutenant who had been his mentor and was trying to get the ammunition off the lorry when they came under attack. "They were lying in salt flats with no cover. The best thing to do is lie down and wait for help but soldiers aren't like that."

He spent six months living in marquees in the Libyan desert carrying out administrative exercises for the British army, was part of the UN deployment in Cyprus and spent considerable time in Northern Ireland.

The opportunity to work with veterans at Erskine just as he became one presented itself as the perfect second career. Aware of the organisation since his childhood in Ayrshire, he says: "I thought it was a very worthwhile cause. It was working with the same people I'd worked with all my life, and it proved to be most enjoyable."

He took up the position of assistant commandant in 1988 when, 72 years after the end of the First World War, there were still 25 veterans of that conflict in the care of Erskine Hospital, a considerable tribute to the quality of care they received. He is in no doubt that Erskine's success was due to the team spirit shared across the entire staff and adds: "The people who really ran it in those days were the nursing staff.

"In the 21st century, as the number of residents who served in the Second World War is dwindling and those who remain are very elderly, inevitably, there has been a change over the years from hospital to care home." In turn that meant the management of funerals and care for bereaved families became a substantial responsibility. With over 100 deaths a year

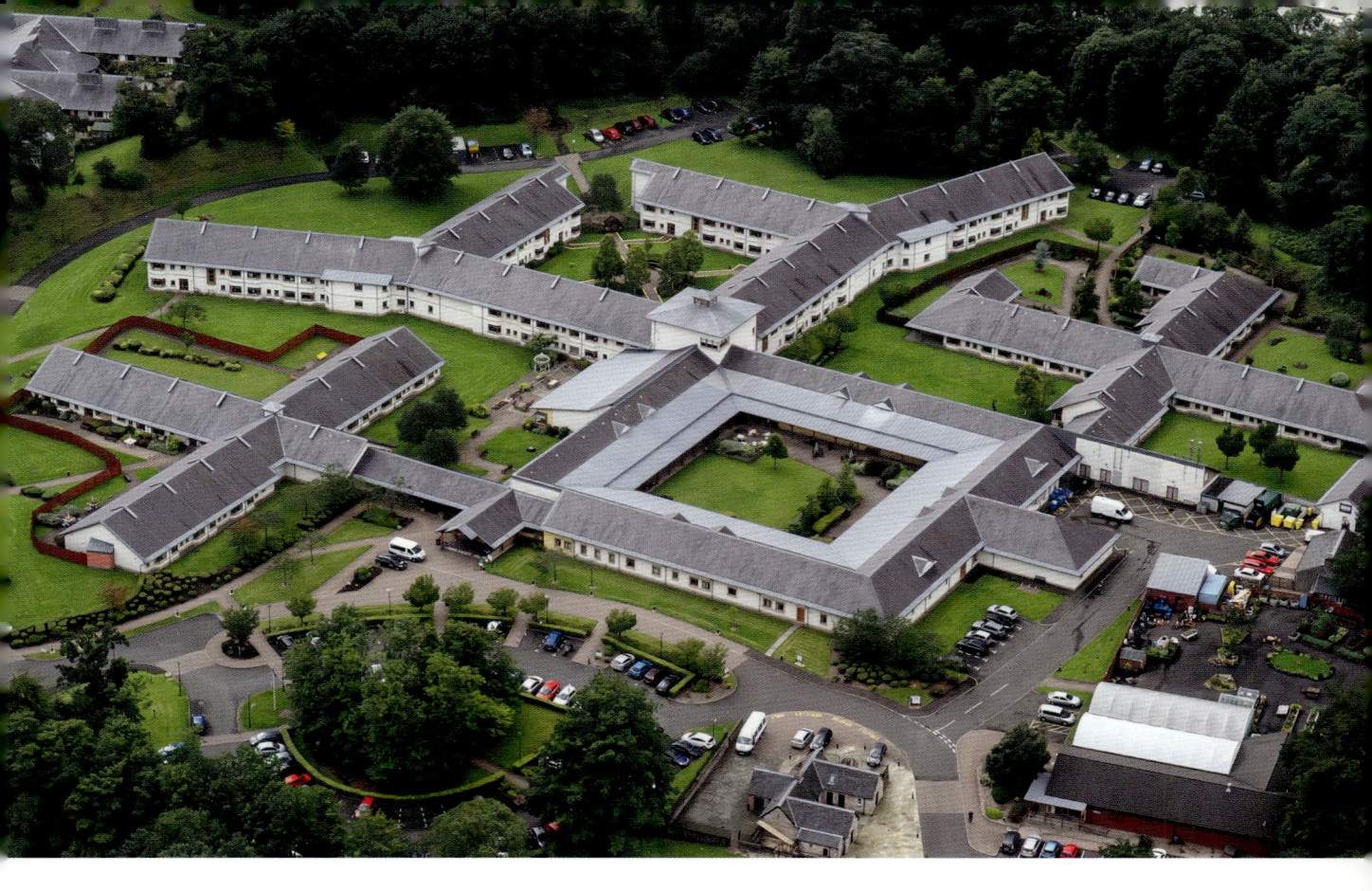

An aerial view of the new Erskine Home complex of linked houses and accessible garden areas.

during his time at the hospital, it was one of his duties as assistant commandant to ensure the highest possible standard of care for dying patients and their families. Although sometimes challenging, it granted him a great deal of satisfaction: "I am proud to have helped people who were bereaved. I've always got a lot of pleasure out of helping people but that is a worthwhile thing that I've done."

Like the residents in his charge, Col Steele lived on the Erskine estate at Bishopton during his time with the charity. He credits the mansion house itself and its parkland surroundings with helping to sustain the legendary community spirit. Like other staff of the time, he recalls with some nostalgia the camaraderie in the long Nightingale wards, where patients were always surrounded by friends and experienced a continuation of the solidarity they had known in the army. He describes it as the opposite of the stereotype of a hospital, "very far from being drab and soulless, with never a dull moment."

Community activities in the games room in the centre of the mansion house included concerts, balls, visits from regimental associations and entertainers. Much as the atmosphere was appreciated by patients, perhaps because it was a haven apart from the increasing bustle and clamour of the late 20th century, the physical buildings and the management structure had become inappropriate. It was no longer required to function as a hospital but fell short of the modern requirements for elderly care.

Col Steele arrived at Erskine to find an organisation living "quite happily" in the past. The matron and the nursing staff all wore traditional uniforms of blue dresses and white head pieces and the managerial positions were structured military ranks. While Erskine wasn't a services-run establishment, it very much felt like being part of the services community, something that the veterans appreciated. "It was very like the army, where you were continually confronted with things you weren't really expecting and that's what made

Colonel Bobby Steele

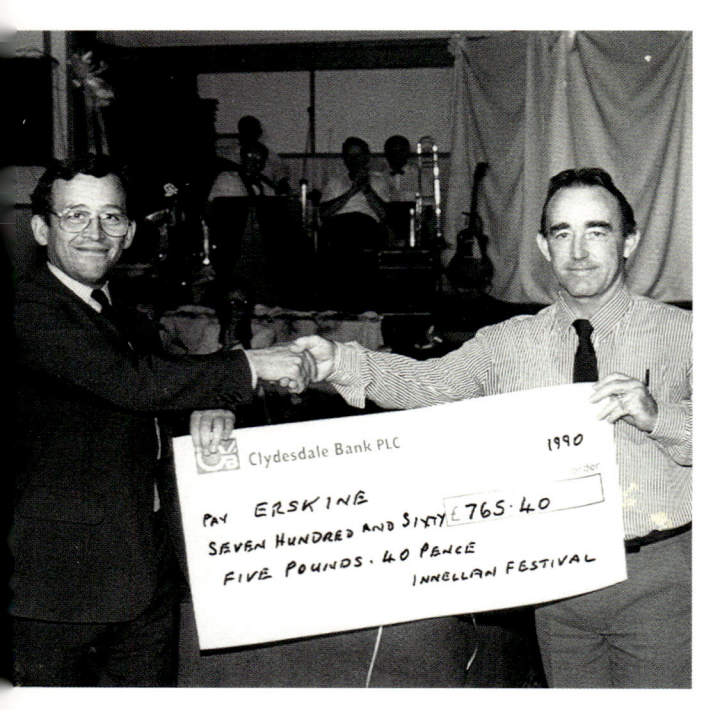

One of Col Steele's enjoyable tasks was to receive cheques from groups which had raised funds.

it so enjoyable. The beauty of Erskine is that we did things our own way. If it had been in the NHS, it would have been just another NHS hospital."

By the 1990s, however, the problems of the outdated facilities, the obsolete equipment and the ever-increasing cost of repairing the fabric of the mansion house could no longer be ignored.

"It was very much early 20th century as opposed to late 20th century. Things really had to change." In 1994, a strategic review committee was charged with examining the hospital's finances, the physical potential and limitations of the existing buildings and how the charity could meet the requirements of new regulations for nursing homes. Its findings were unequivocal: however much was spent on refurbishing and additional facilities, the hospital would not be registered as a nursing home and would therefore lose all public funding. Without payments on behalf of patients through the NHS, social security or social work departments, Erskine would not be able to make ends meet.

There was only one solution: to build new facilities and move out of the money-draining mansion house. It was a complex, logistical challenge made even more difficult by the enormous emotional attachment the residents had to the old building. He dismisses the idea that planning the move must have used his expertise in military transport and supply chains. "We followed the best way with such matters which was to sit down in the business room of the old mansion house over coffee and biscuits and make a note of how people wanted to do it and the nurses and staff did a very good job."

The initial resistance on the part of many of the veterans was overcome by the family atmosphere which galvanised the community into saying: "We have to rebuild this place."

That aim was fulfilled in 2000 with the move to the new Erskine Home, which remains the flagship building. The day of the move was an emotional, bittersweet affair, as veterans were taken in wheelchairs onto buses and driven up the road to the new facilities. Of course their arrival was greeted with cheers. Such moments embody the spirit of solidarity and determination at Erskine for Bobby Steele: "Moving the hospital up the road was something I've always been proud of on behalf of the staff who embodied that old 'will-do' attitude: it had to be done, so they did it."

With equal pride, he points out that throughout the radical changes over the decades the core mission of the organisation, to provide care for the ex-service personnel, has never altered. The need for surgery and rehabilitation for those who lost limbs in the First World War became the need to care for them in old age. Later casualties have suffered from post-traumatic stress as a result of their experiences. For them, too, the Erskine spirit has provided healing. "One of the important things for anybody who suffers from PTSD is being in a community where people understand what the problem is. Half the battle is being able to talk to people who understand. It is especially important once people have left the services because they can't do what we would do on active service: go down to the NAAFI, have a drink and talk about it. I remember interviewing Bill McDowall, who had been in the Falklands, to see if he would be suitable for a house at Erskine. I was chatting just to get to know him and it was the usual thing of swapping experiences. I thought no more about it but he told me later that simple talk had been of great help to him. There weren't many people with PTSD at Erskine but sharing experience is always helpful." He also firmly believes that being able to contribute towards the place that has given them a home through gardening or being taken on to the staff instils a sense of purpose.

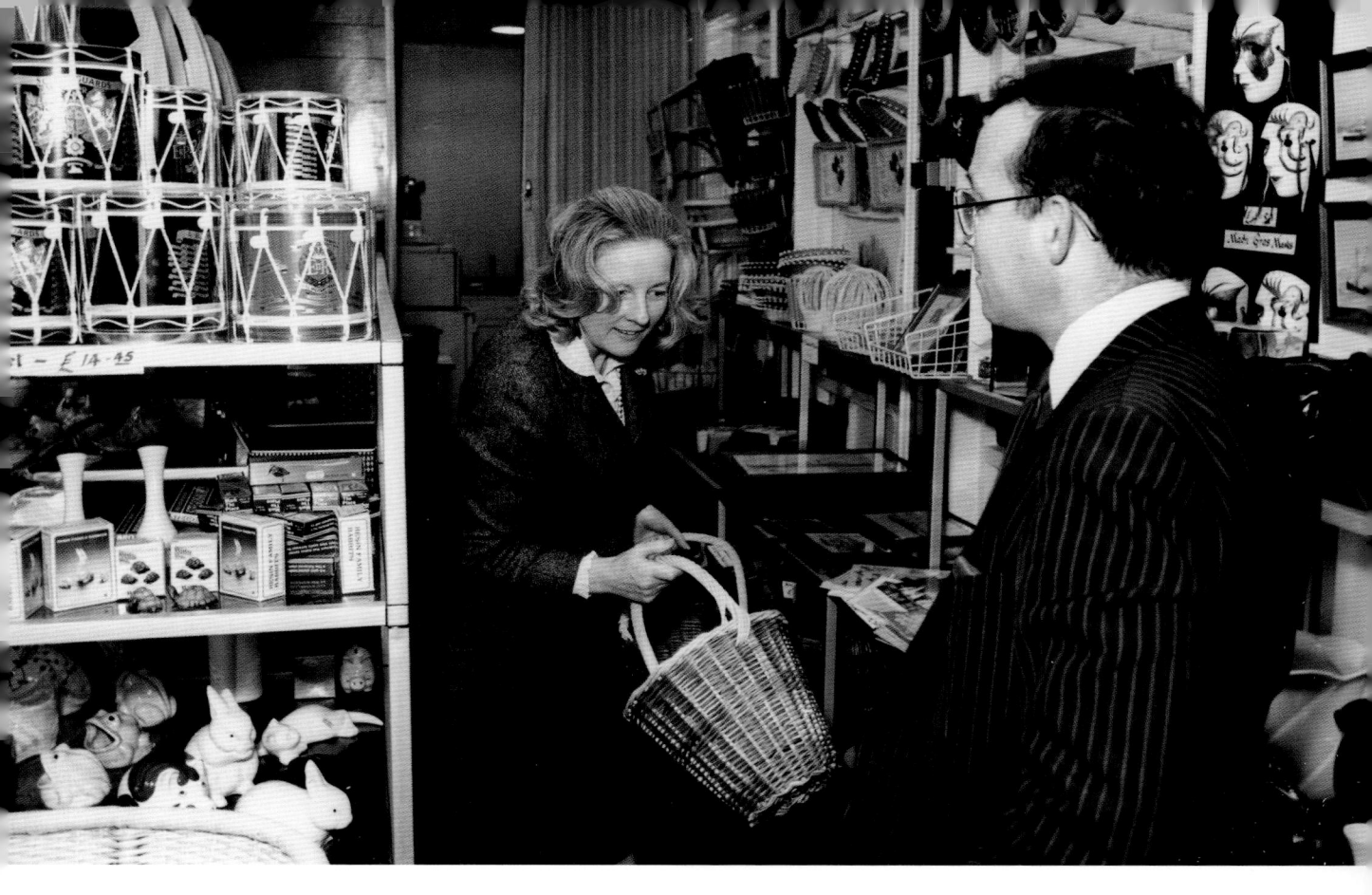

His life still centres round the military, as does that of his brother. Bobby is now Area Secretary West for the Royal Regiment of Scotland and manager of the Royal Highland Fusiliers Museum in Glasgow. David is one of 13 Military Knights of Windsor, historically known as the Poor Knights of Windsor as a result of having to pay a ransom to gain their freedom after the Crusades, but now retired officers who receive lodgings at Windsor Castle in return for providing an escort for the Order of the Garter.

Bobby retains great admiration for the veterans that he met at Erskine. "The great thing about Erskine for me was that I met a lot of very fascinating people. Just because someone is old, it doesn't mean to say they lose the characteristics they had when they were young. Stories you hear from them are quite remarkable yet very matter of fact. There was no question that anybody thought there was anything special that had happened to them. Whether they had been Japanese prisoners of war, lost in no man's land, or left for dead on the battlefield, that's just the way it was and they got on with it."

That such sacrifice continues, often unappreciated, makes it crucial that organisations like Erskine continue to exist and flourish, he says. "Some people don't appreciate how nasty the world we live in can be sometimes. We must look after our veterans. They do a very good job for our country, one not fully understood by people who don't know what they're talking about. One of the lessons Erskine has learned is to try and develop that process of looking after old and young. Progress has to continue. And it is important that we look after our veterans." There is a chuckle, followed by: "Well, I would say that, wouldn't I? Because I'm one myself."

The Erskine shop in Glasgow sold goods made in the workshops.

Bill McDowall

"If I hadn't found Erskine, I wouldn't be here now. I can't praise it highly enough."

Bill McDowall had just turned 16 when he reported for duty at the Guards' depot at Pirbright, in Surrey, to start a year's training. Very quickly, he found himself stationed in Belfast. "That was an eye-opener in so many different ways. Everything in Northern Ireland, especially in a city like Belfast, was so normal to somebody from the west of Scotland. The accents are different, yes, but other things – the shops, the way people dressed, people's attitudes towards such things as Catholic-Protestant, Rangers-Celtic, was so normal, and yet the environment you found yourself in was completely alien.

"I'd been to Belfast as a kid, to visit family, and I had been brought up in the Orange Lodge. That was the side of the story we knew but you realise that there are two sides to every story. I think a lot of soldiers from the west of Scotland got off the train or ferry in Northern Ireland with a preconception of what they were going to do. You realise that is only one side of the story, that life is a collection of grey areas and that very, very few things in life are in black and white.

"We were involved in a couple of riot situations, which were frightening. It's difficult to explain what it feels like when you're standing there and there's maybe 15 of you with riot shields on the baseline and maybe another 30 military and RUC personnel behind you, and you've got what looks like a million people in front of you, although it is actually between 100 and 150.

"When they're charging at you, throwing paving slabs, petrol bombs or glass marbles from slings, the thought that goes through your head is: what happens when the baseline collapses? That's where all your training kicks in, that's where you rely on the guy to your right and the guy to your left to hold his space.

"For four-and-a-half months you basically lived off your nerves. When you walked out of the gate on patrol you'd do a 'hard target': you wouldn't walk out, you would run, and the guys in the armoured guard posts would cover you. I spent my time walking backwards on patrols, because I was the tail-end Charlie. I'd be watching the backs of the other three members of my patrol.

"I still remember the first time somebody called me a British bastard and spat at me. We used to do pub checks at 11pm. The natives were definitely hostile. They'd shout, 'We know where your family lives'. When you're 18 or 19 and feel that kind of hate being directed at you, you'd think: 'I've not done anything: I don't want to do anything to you'. You could see the hatred in their eyes. It was a hatred for you and what you represented. I can understand that they saw us as the tools of the oppressor. I'm 54 now and can look back and say, that's what it was. But at that time, on the ground, I started to hate them back. You realise their hatred was generational."

He was 20, recently married with a young son, when the Argentinians seized the Falkland Islands in April 1982. The 20,000-strong Task Force included the 2nd Battalion

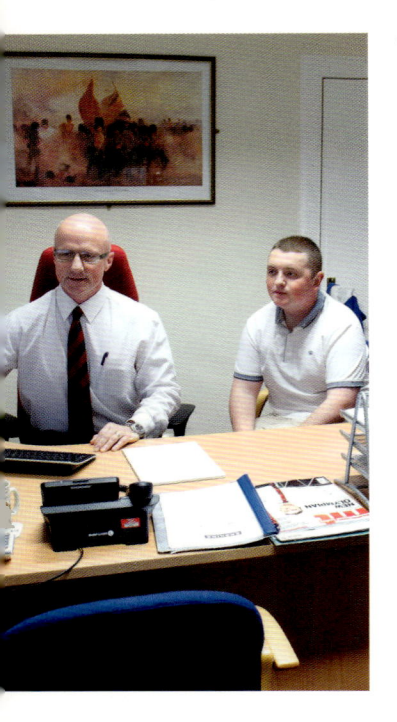

At work in the IT office, Bill McDowall has a vital role in the running of Erskine.

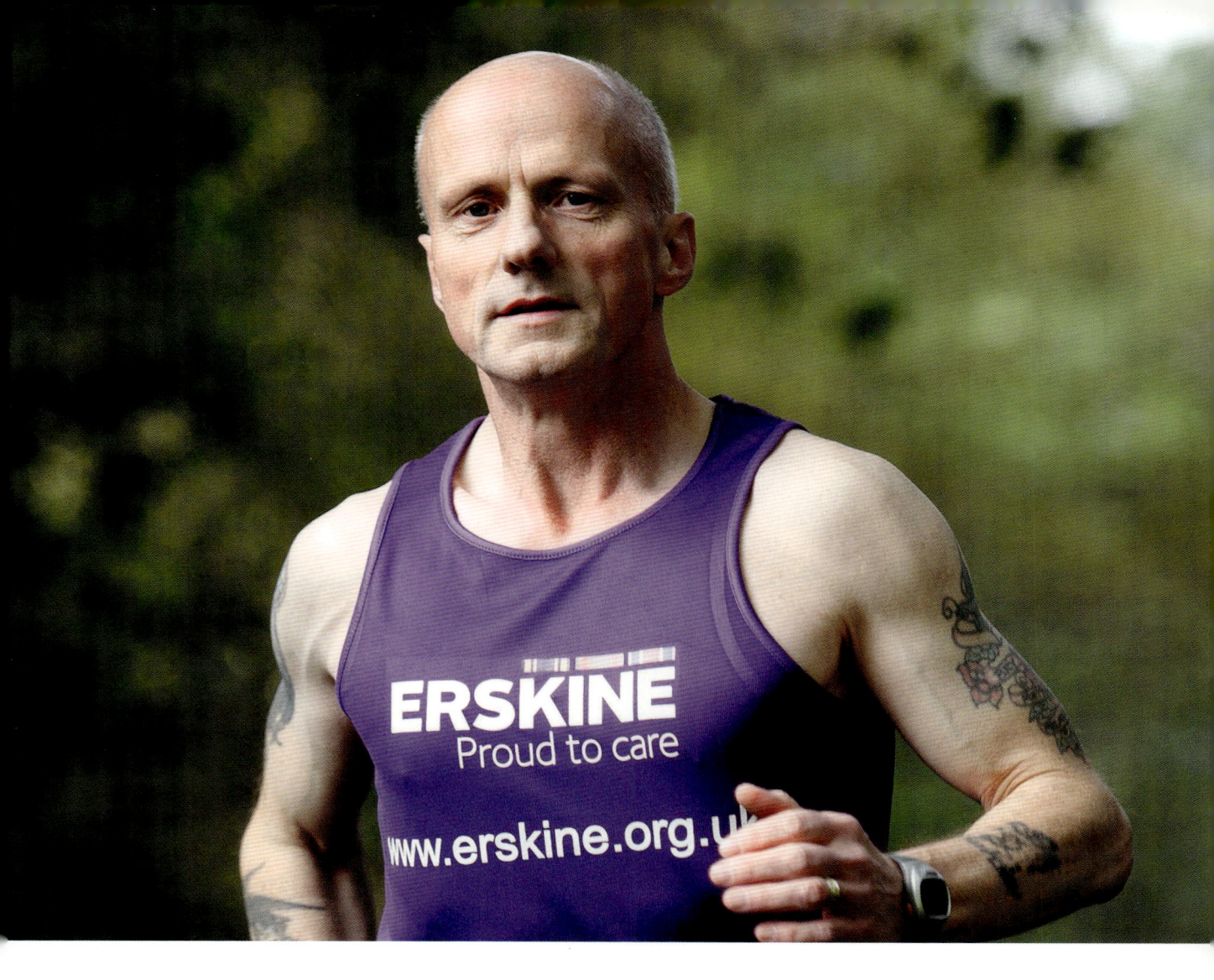

Scots Guards. They landed at Fitzroy on June 6 with the objective of taking the heavily defended Mount Tumbledown. "The only thing we knew, moving into Tumbledown, was that we were doing Advance to Contact. We weren't going out on patrol as we'd done in Northern Ireland, where something might happen. We knew there were Argentine marines on Tumbledown. We knew they were elite troops, that they were well-armed, well-fed and had had three months to dig in. And they were in front of us.

"We knew the order would come for us to get out of our little trenches and walk forward and keep walking until we made contact with them. We had been crouching in our wee trench, sharing our last weak beef drink between three of us. On average each guy probably had about 60 rounds of ammunition. The problem for the British army in the Falklands was the supply line. When we heard about the Atlantic Conveyor being sunk, we knew it took a lot of our supplies with it.

"We'd been reliably told that some Argentine snipers had been equipped with American-made night-sights. We hadn't. We had one night-sight, some phosphorus grenades and some high-explosive grenades."

In the final battle for Tumbledown, the battalion came under heavy machine-gun fire. Bill lost nine comrades. "I still find it difficult to talk about the moments that changed my life forever. I was confused, scared and a long way from home." Lying in waterlogged trenches

Bill's gratitude to Erskine has inspired him to take part in fundraising challenges.

Bill McDowall

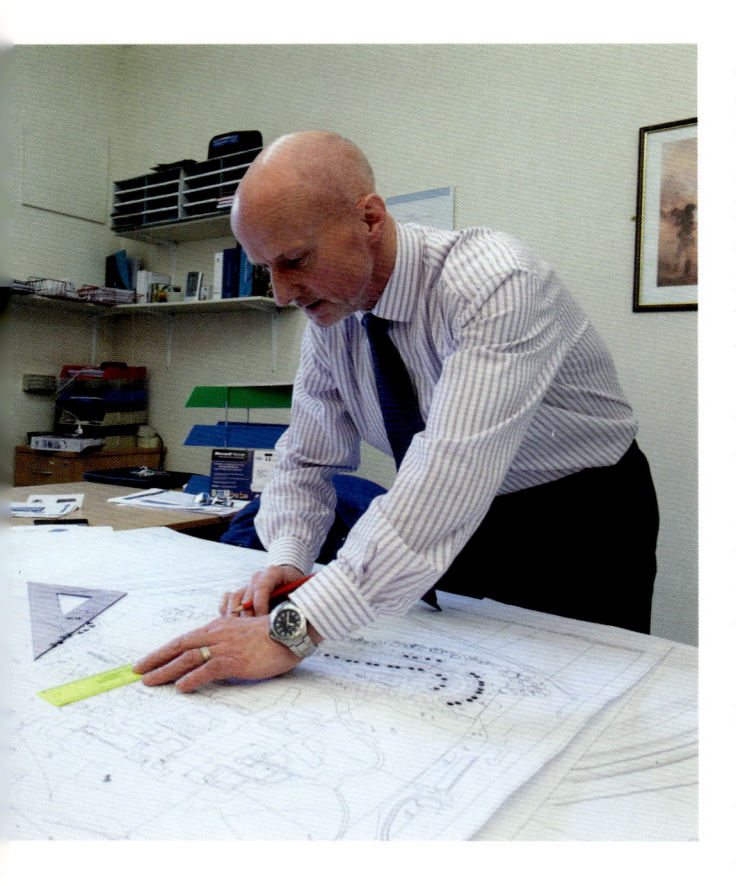

Bill hard at work.

alongside his fellow Scots Guards, waiting for the command to start moving forward, fear was kept at bay with bravado. "You're glad it's so cold, because then you could blame your shaking on the cold … You think, when the contact finally happens, I hope it's not me. I don't want it to be somebody else, but I don't want it to be me." Inside his jacket he had a photograph of his wife and young son. "All I could think of was, I just want to get home. I don't want to be here. That wasn't a coward talking. I just wanted to be home."

The attacks on the Sir Galahad and the Sir Tristram with the loss of 51 lives, had taken place two days earlier on June 8. We got credited with shooting down three Argentine jets. I remember the jets came flying down and people running around shouting, 'early morning raid!' but the jets were past us before anyone could react. We could see the explosions in the bay, where the troopships Sir Galahad and Sir Tristram, were anchored. Everybody was running around shouting, 'They're bombing ships, Sir the ships!' The jets came back for a second run onto Bluff Cove. We were dug in on the hills. This time we were ready for them. I kept my fingers on my Browning machine-gun and my number two kept feeding the belt in. We kept hammering everything we could at these jets. The first jet tried to bank away but its whole underside was visible.

"For a fraction of a second you're thinking you're shooting this target which is a plane and you suddenly realise there's a person sitting there. And you get that feeling of – 'that's a human being, not a nameless, faceless person but a father or a son'. A few minutes later, we were running down the hill at full speed into the water at Bluff Cove to meet what was left of the Welsh Guards coming out of the water. I was waist-deep in the water, trying to help get them into the life-rafts. Guys are screaming for help but you don't know where to touch them. Everywhere you touched hurt.

"They were fellow Guardsmen, fellow soldiers. A couple of days earlier, we had spent up to eight hours on the landing-craft and you think: 'that could have been us'. You're glad it's not, then you realise this is the end-result of what we're here for. This isn't a training exercise. People are dying and others are going to die. As a soldier, all you can do is hope that the next time, if it is your turn, it doesn't hurt too much."

The Scots Guards took Mount Tumbledown, almost 12 hours after leaving their start-line. On June 14, the Argentinians surrendered at Port Stanley.

Having secured his deepest wish to return home to his family, Bill had to face a different but equally fraught challenge. To civilians in Britain, the Falklands War had resulted in some terrible casualties but had been mercifully brief. It had touched most peoples' lives only through television images. For Bill, the inescapable images were much darker and recurring. Adjustment to others' petty concerns about the price of beer or the scheduling of Coronation Street was near impossible. "I came close to losing my grip on reality because I could not understand how everybody's life was so normal," he says. He had a lot of mixed feelings, including guilt. "There really were times when I wanted to grab people and ask them, 'Do you understand what I've seen? Do you know what I've done?" With hindsight, it is clear he was suffering from post-traumatic stress disorder. That diagnosis, however, lay many years into the future. He was diagnosed with osteoarthritis. It was a shock when that resulted in medical discharge from the Scots Guards in 1986. He and Beverley by this time had two young children. They lost their army accommodation and found themselves homeless and unemployed in west London.

"We spent ages on the move. We were in run-down bed-and-breakfasts, one place after another." There were times when they had to be out of their room by 7.30am. They weren't allowed back in until 7pm, which meant they had to sit in their car someplace. The family was eventually given a one-bed flat in a tough part of the city.

Bill had no skills apart from those he'd learned in the Army and no prospect of a job. It was the start of a painful, difficult decade. He suffered so seriously from depression that he was admitted to a psychiatric unit for a while. Then he suffered a heart attack. It is hardly surprising that he considered taking his own life.

"I just couldn't see a way out of the situation I was in and felt I was bringing my family down with me. My life was completely out of control. I was almost living like a recluse. My marriage was virtually on the rocks. I was drinking a lot and felt my life had been absolutely ruined."

In 1996 the McDowalls moved to Bill's home town of Greenock. He learned from the benefits office that he was eligible for a war pension. Shamefully, this had never been explained to him. But the pension could not be backdated, although he had lost out on nearly 10 years' worth of payments.

There was one stroke of good fortune, however. "Mary Morgan, a fantastic woman from the War Pensions Agency, was amazing. She encouraged me to speak to my GP and I was able to speak to psychiatrists and other experts about my experiences." He was eventually diagnosed with PTSD and was also put in touch with Erskine. "It was like a breath of fresh air. It immediately felt just right. You could talk to people here, talk to them about anything and you felt they understood you.

"It was also genuinely humbling to be able to meet some of the veterans of the First World War. Their stories were truly remarkable. It put my own life into perspective."

Erskine was able to offer the family a cottage on the Bishopton estate. "Everything seemed to change for us that day. Before I came here I had been very withdrawn but I got a job here, and in time I began to feel that I was really part of something worthwhile."

He has been convinced of that now for decades. With Erskine's support, he undertook a computing course at James Watt College. It led to his being appointed as Erskine's IT manager – a vital role in the organisation he fulfils to this day.

His gratitude to Erskine and the positive impact it had on his life has resulted in him often being the public face of the charity for fundraising events. His story, however, is a reminder that those who are willing to go into combat to protect the rest of us are owed a duty of care. As Bill puts it: "There are an awful lot of servicemen and women out there who need the help that only somewhere like Erskine provides."

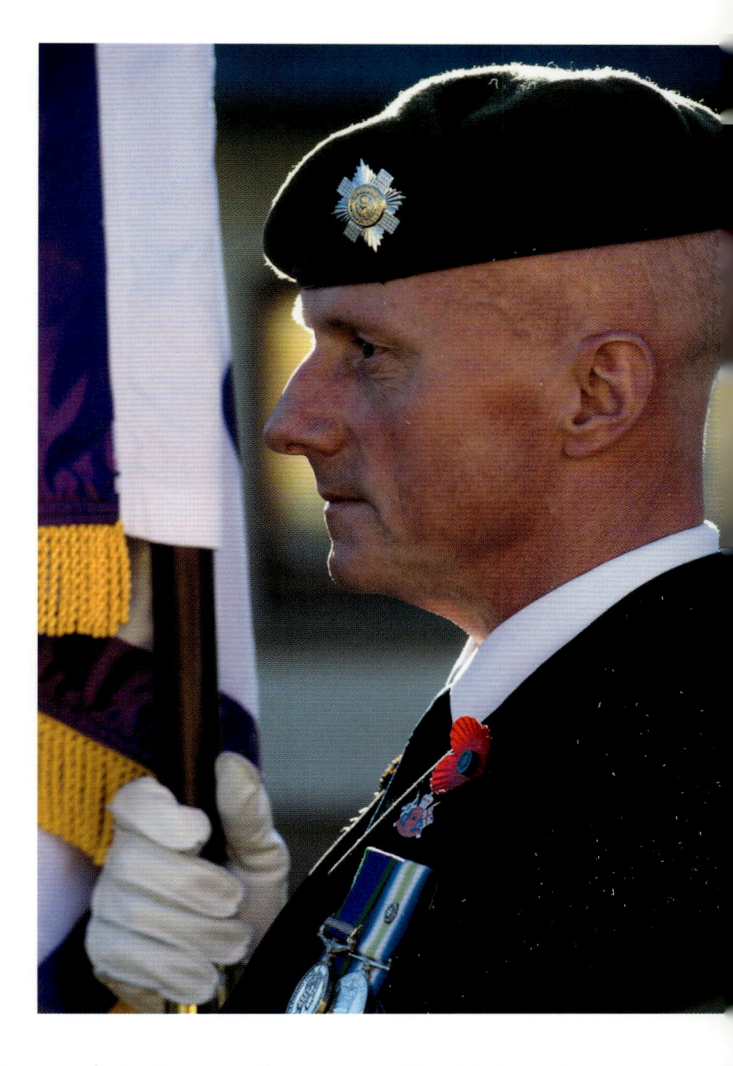

In addition to being a veteran and Erskine's IT manager, Bill is honoured and proud to be the Erskine standard bearer.

Three Generations of Caring

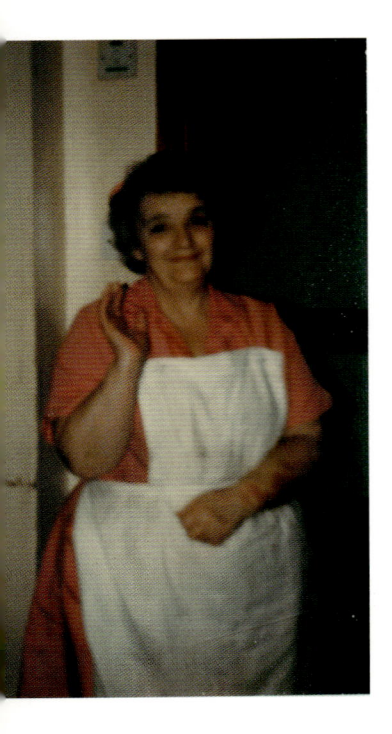

Jean Jones: always a cheering presence in the old Nightingale wards.

"Some of the older residents tell me they remember my Gran and they like that continuity. Erskine is a family."
Karen Findlay, nurse, third generation of her family to work at Erskine.

There are certain skills, trades and professions that run in families. Military service is an obvious one but the Erskine story shows that caring for veterans can also flow down through the generations. Residents and staff describe Erskine as having a family spirit, referring to its caring ethos. The Jones family interprets it more literally. Four of its members are currently on the staff, with others having worked there in the past. Their experiences over more than four decades mirror the changes at Erskine from hospital and rehabilitation unit to nursing and care homes, mainly for the elderly.

Jean Jones was keen to work at Erskine Hospital after moving with her growing family to Erskine New Town in the 1970s. Laughing, she says: "The first time I went into the old hospital, the smell of urine caught the back of my throat and I thought I would never stick working there." She stayed for more than 30 years, a length of service that is not unusual, retiring at 67 in 1997.

There were several very elderly veterans from the First World War when she started as a cleaner, then known as orderlies. From the beginning her morning routine never varied: "I would walk down the ward in the main building and I would say 'Good Morning' to every old man and go back up the other side and greet each one." It's not surprising that the patients referred to her as the salt of the earth but she could also deliver a reprimand if necessary. One elderly gent who was a habitual complainer would be sharply reminded of his good fortune in having all his needs taken care of "with no need to pay income tax." It's an example of the way she regarded talking to the patients as an integral part of her job and while she could mete out the occasional scolding, she had sincere respect for the veterans and genuinely enjoyed providing cups of tea or slices of toast and the occasional egg boiled to precise liking. "Those old men fought for us, to give us our freedom to live in a country with no dictators. You could get a real history lesson from talking to them.

"One had been a prisoner of war in Japan and he used to walk endlessly up and down. It must have been a terrible experience. I got on very well with another, who had fought with the Gurkhas and there was one who was grumpy but liked me to sit and talk. I liked all of them. There was a lovely atmosphere with these old men. I loved it."

Her respect for the ex-servicemen was widely shared. She recalls fondly that the old mansion building positioned on the south bank of the Clyde gave the residents an uninterrupted view of ships, which would sound their horns in salute when they passed what was still described as a hospital for limbless ex-servicemen. A similar spirit inspired the volunteers who played a huge part in the social life of the institution. Jean particularly remembers one group taking the old soldiers off in a coach every Saturday. "They loved it, they used to be sitting waiting at the front door every week. The people who ran the bus were getting old themselves and had to stop but they ended with a great big party for the soldiers."

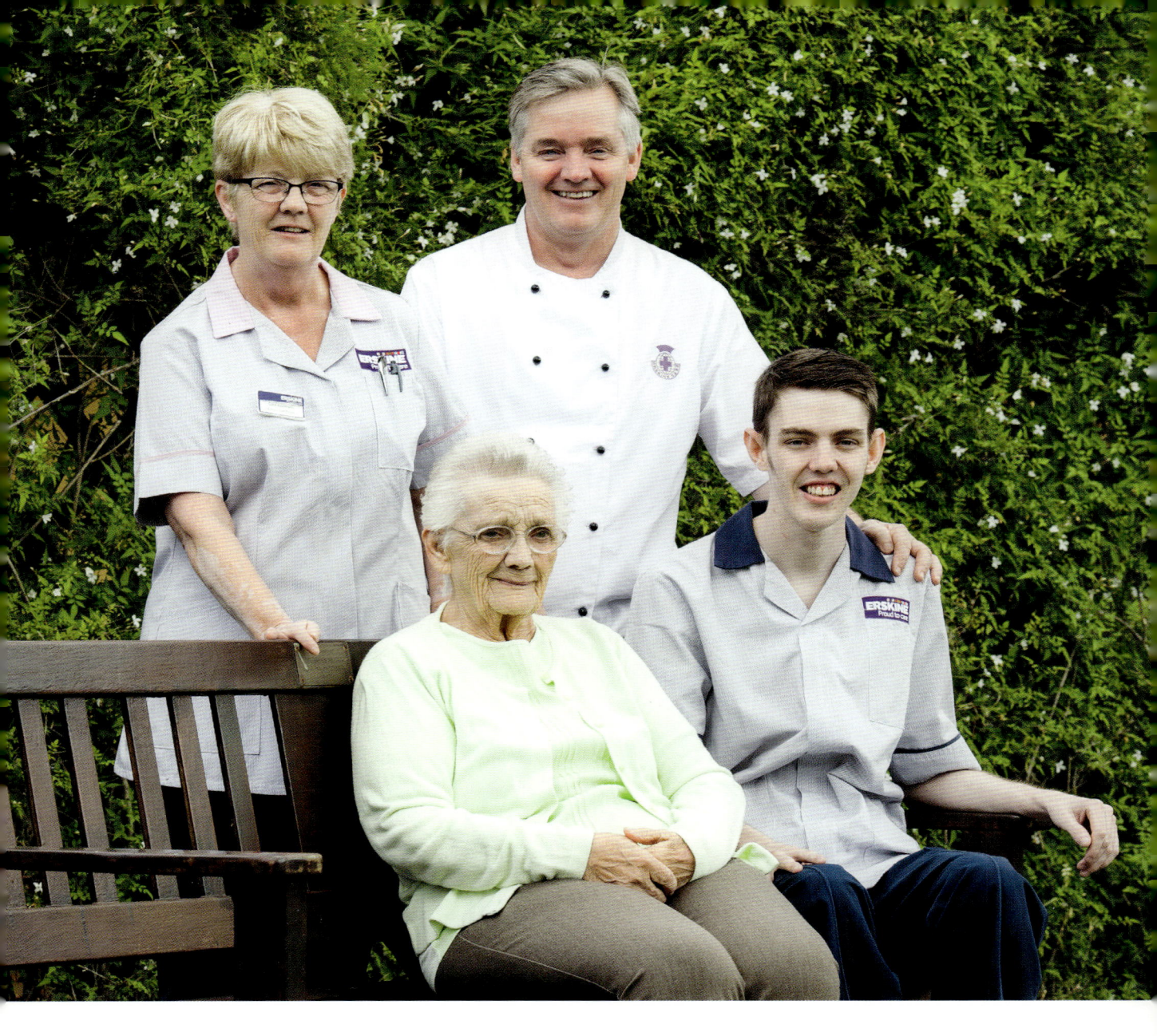

She understood something of army life because her husband, David, had been in the army, as a dispatch rider. It was his unfailing insistence on courtesy to all, something all their 12 children learned at an early age, that prompted her personal greeting for each patient. They did not know that, with her husband confined to bed in his later years, Jean would do an extra caring shift when she got home from work.

One of their daughters, Eileen Gardiner, is a care assistant, who has herself received a long-service award for more than 30 years at Erskine. She initially took up the job when her two daughters were very young because she could work an evening shift from 5pm to 9pm enabling her to share childcare with her husband. Later she moved on to nightshift and then to dayshift.

Erskine has gone through a transformation in her time. The needs of veterans had

A family of carers: (from left to right) Eileen, care assistant; Jean, domestic orderly; Michael, chef; Matthew, care assistant.

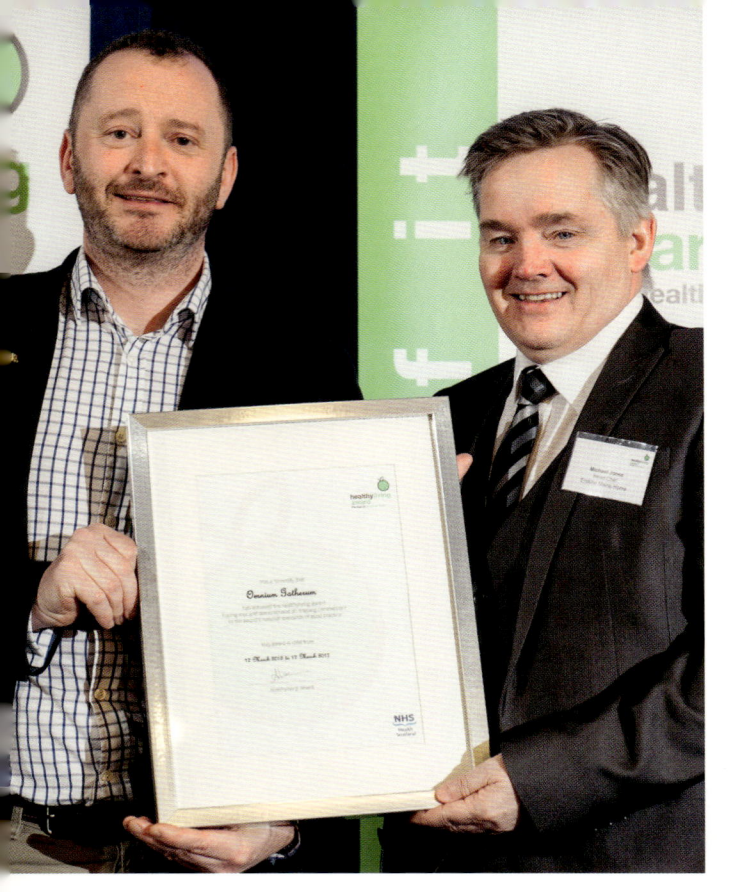

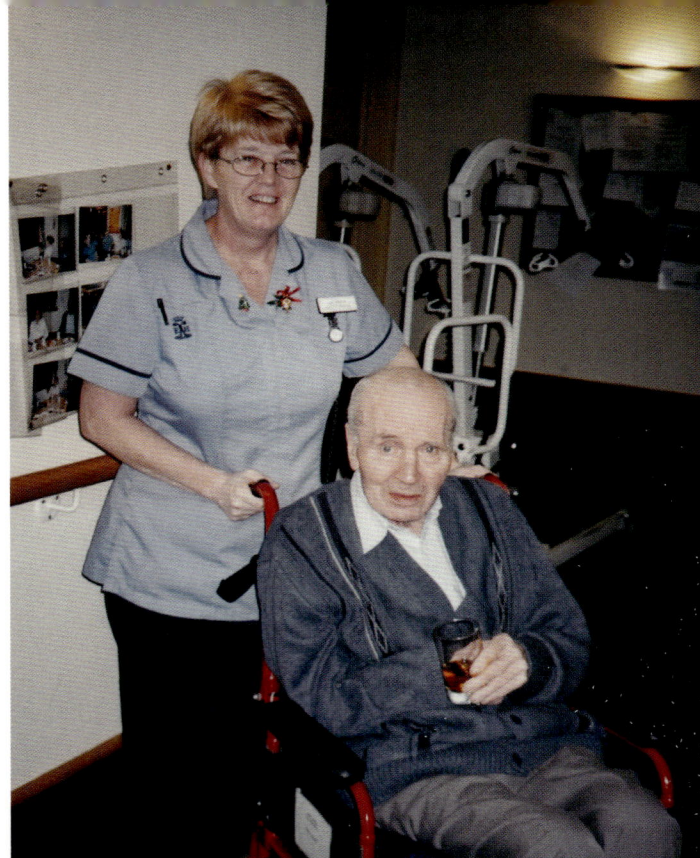

Above: Michael Jones receives the healthy living award in 2015.

Above right: Eileen with veteran from the Red Cross House in The Erskine Home.

changed from the original focus of providing artificial limbs and a healing environment for those who had lost arms and legs in the First World War. Healthcare needs changed as Erskine increasingly admitted ex-service personnel who had become ill in later years or needed care in old age. A grand mansion converted into a hospital in the early part of the 20th century with additional buildings added on an ad hoc basis was unable to meet the very different needs of the 21st century yet soaked up financial resources.

The new Erskine Home, opened in 2000, replacing the old hospital wards with purpose-built accommodation and providing a single room for every resident. It was an enormous step forward in comfort, hygiene and privacy. Jean, remembering the camaraderie and the jokes among the residents of her day, wonders whether a little sociability has been lost. For Eileen, however, the physical improvements have ushered in an era of other welcome changes. "We used to have to wear a blue overall with a white apron and a starched hat. Now we wear trousers and a tunic, which is a lot more practical, especially when you have to reach over someone."

There have been significant changes in the type of residents over the years. These include the admission of women, not only those who had been in the services but spouses of veterans. Inevitably, as in the general population, there has been a great increase in elderly residents suffering from dementia, requiring staff to be aware of the need to keep track of the movements of some residents.

The Jones family is not the only one to have several members at Erskine. Jean Jones' recollection that Maureen Lundie, the matron, had two daughters who also worked there, sparks a series of names of old colleagues for whom Erskine was a family calling. The sense of community is reinforced by the fact that the charity has always been a major employer for the local area.

Jean's son, Michael, began as a kitchen porter at Erskine in 1979, when he left school.

One consequence of the very low staff turnover is that not only do the residents grow older, so do the staff. As a result of the hospital being a converted mansion, the kitchens were a long way from the wards. "At the time the person in charge of the kitchen porters kept asking if he could have some younger staff," said Michael, who, as a teenager, fitted the bill for hauling heavy trolleys. He also began to help the head chef and gradually acquired kitchen skills, working his way up to head chef and then catering manager at the old hospital.

With the move to new buildings, he became head chef at Erskine Mains Home, a satellite home in the town of Erskine. The change gave him far greater contact with the residents. Instead of dispatching food to distant wards and only meeting residents in the passing, he served up within sight of the dining room. It has given him a new impetus to provide appetising, healthy food for the residents. He has already garnered a number of awards for "going the extra mile" in food safety, always essential in catering but the priority when preparing meals for the elderly. With a Healthy Living Award also under his belt, he's aiming for the next level in the scheme promoted by the NHS in Scotland. "It's a bit of a challenge but we have reduced salt, sugar and fat in all our dishes without any complaints – although someone in their 90s is not concerned about reducing salt and they will add it to their food at the table. We have provided more choice on the menu. Here, macaroni cheese is a healthy option because we don't add butter to the sauce and use skimmed milk and low-fat cheese. We have introduced a fruit bar so that there is always fresh fruit available when they have tea or coffee throughout the day." Even that is not simple as it sounds. Biting into fruit can be a problem for the residents, so it is soft fruit or served cut into pieces. That rules out apples, because they discolour so quickly and can also be a choking hazard but kiwi fruit and grapes have proved popular. Offering tasty food that elderly mouths and digestive systems can handle is Michael's stock-in-trade. "If steak pie is a problem, for instance, we can blend the steak and they will still enjoy the taste."

Having spent his entire working life at Erskine, Michael says he has never wanted to work anywhere else. All the residents in the 34-bed Erskine Mains Home address him as "Chef" and, as he heads towards 40 years' service to the charity, it's clear that he not only enjoys the challenges of cooking for the elderly, but relishes interacting with them, just as his mother did.

Even more extraordinary is that two of Michael's brothers and a sister were also members of the Erskine team for several years and one of his sons, Matthew, is now a care assistant.

Also among the third generation of her family to work at Erskine is Karen Findlay, the daughter of Eileen Gardiner and granddaughter of Jean Jones. From an early age, she wanted to be a nurse but began her working life in retail. The responsibilities of motherhood, however, made the shift patterns at the Erskine Home attractive and she began work as a care assistant in 2008. She enjoyed it so much that she decided to fulfil her girlhood dream and train as a nurse. With a degree in nursing from the University of the West of Scotland, she continues to work at Erskine because she likes caring for older people and says: "Although it is no longer a hospital, I can still use my nursing skills because the residents have different medical conditions, long-term illnesses or pain." That job satisfaction would be found in almost any branch of nursing but for Karen, there's an extra family dimension. "Some of the older residents tell me they remember my Gran and they like that continuity. Erskine is a family." The future is unknowable but, with Karen's two young daughters saying they want to be nurses, Erskine might yet benefit from a fourth generation with the caring gene.

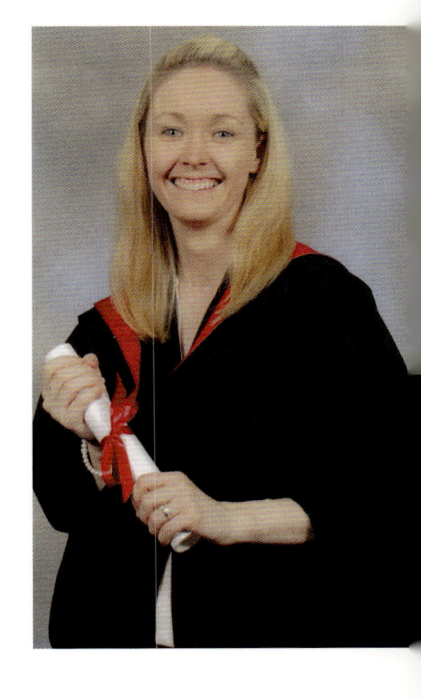

Karen Findlay graduated with a degree in Nursing in 2015.

Three Generations of Caring

From Superintendent to Commandant to Chief Executive

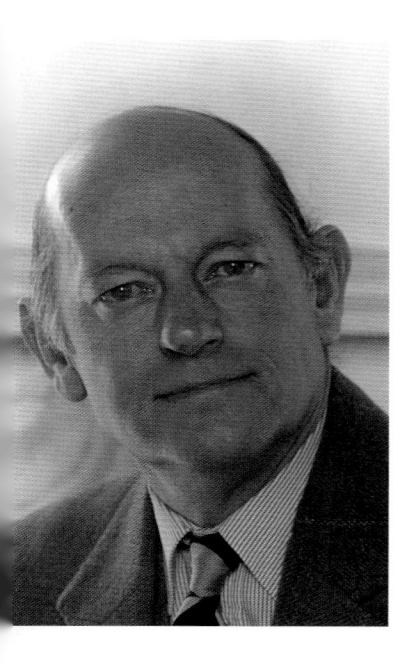

Colonel Ken Sheperd.

"The bottom line is that we are here to care for those men and women who put their lives on the line for their country, or were prepared to. Many of them had friends who made the ultimate sacrifice and this is as true today as it was at the end of the Second World War." Colonel Martin Gibson, chief executive at Erskine from 1995 to 2009.

The day-to-day running of the hospital has always been carried out by a military officer. There have been ten, since 1916, when Lieutenant J Napier was appointed superintendent. It was perhaps significant that the second holder of that post, Colonel C A Gourlay, was a physician, since he was appointed in 1928, after the death of Sir William Macewen in 1924. With the last of the superintendents, Captain John Wentworth Farquhar, the role went to a former naval officer for the first time. As captain of HMS Diomede, he had intercepted the German passenger/cargo ship SS Idarwald off Cape Corrientes, Cuba on December 8 and 9, 1940. Before the ship could be captured, however, the German crew scuttled their ship set fire to her and took to their boats. The crew of Diomede fought the fire and took the Idarwald in tow but she had to be cast off shortly afterwards and sank.

He took over at Erskine in 1950 and is recalled as delegating much of the daily running of the hospital to his assistants and the healthcare side of things to the then matron, Mary Cameron, known for both a very strict regime and a kind heart.

His successor, Colonel David Boyle, who had served with the Argyll and Sutherland Highlanders, had a close bond with the veterans, strengthened by his wartime experience as a prisoner of war of the Japanese in the camp at Tamarkan, the story of which was made famous in the film Bridge over the River Kwai. Former colleagues recall him as devoted to the wellbeing of the men in his care, to the point where he had few outside interests other than a passion for golf. That was more than matched, however, by his dedication to Erskine and particularly to fundraising at a time when new income was desperately needed. He established the idea of Friends of Erskine, where community groups would hold events to raise money and made strong links with local schools. He and his wife lived in a house on the estate and, along with their pet dog, were very much part of the hospital community, making his sudden death in 1983 a severe shock.

Colonel Ken Shepherd, who took over later that year, after serving with the Royal Highland Fusiliers, was a quiet figure by comparison. He ran the hospital in a collegiate way, involving the two assistant commandants, medical officer and matron in major decisions. It was an approach that paved the way for senior staff to participate in the strategic review of the existing buildings and the future development of patient care set up in 1993, two years before the end of his stint as commandant. Once it was clear that even extensive refurbishment and additions to the existing buildings would not meet the regulations for registration as a nursing home, the decision was taken to build new facilities in the extensive

Colonel David Boyle.

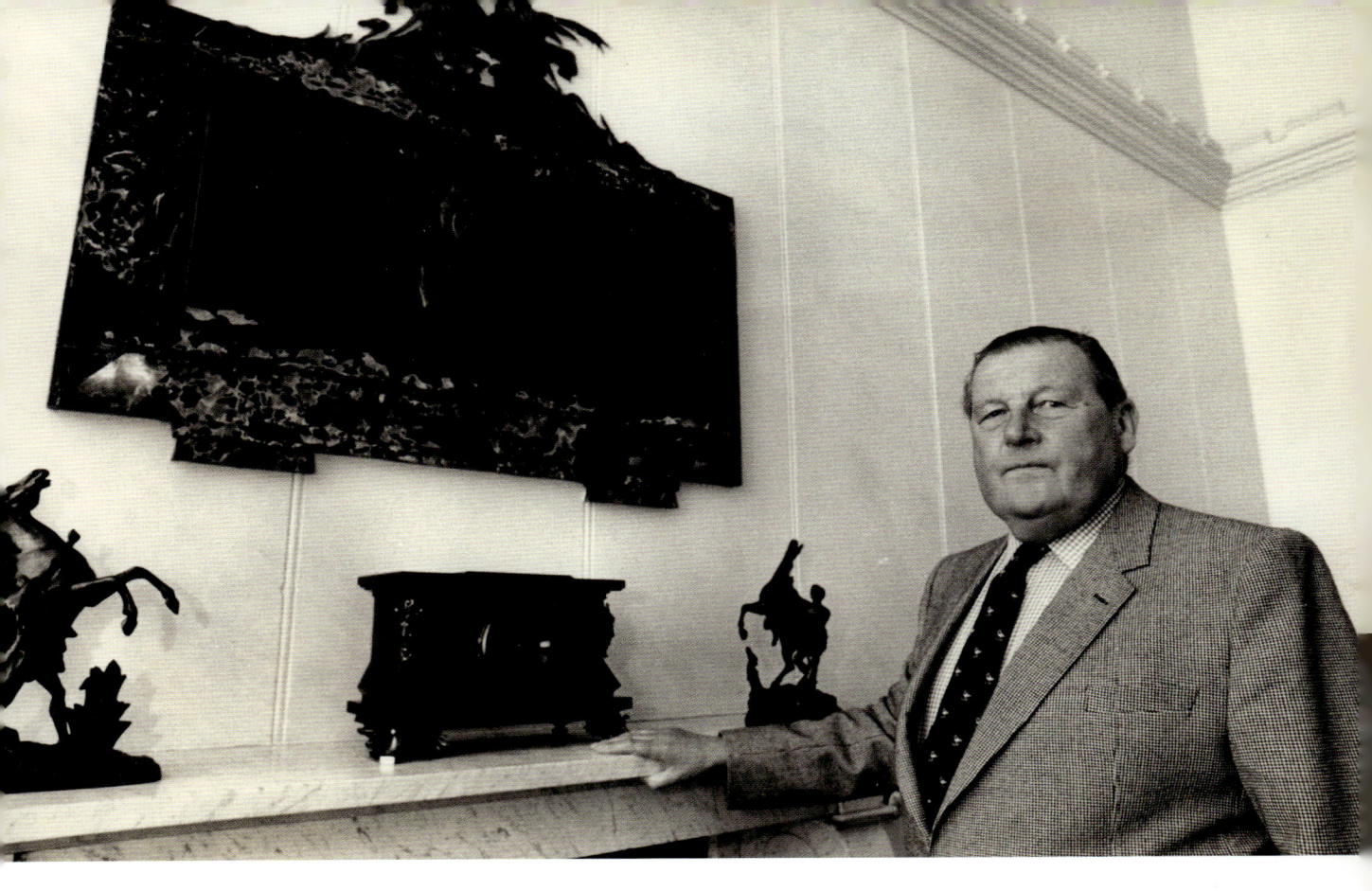

grounds but also to establish sister-homes elsewhere to allow veterans in other parts of Scotland to benefit from Erskine's care.

Colonel Martin Gibson, moved from being Chief of Staff of the Army in Scotland to chief executive of the hospital in 1995. That it was still referred to as Erskine Hospital, even occasionally as the Princess Louise Scottish Hospital, although most of its patients were elderly and in need of day-to-day care rather than surgery, was an indication of just how out of date some aspects were.

When he arrived, there were four residents who had served in the First World War, 77 years after the end of that conflict, a testament to the care they had received. "One could describe being in a trench with horse-drawn gun carriages going over the top of him. Imagine what that must feel like. I had the privilege of sharing their experiences that were the foundation of Erskine and it allowed me to relate to that."

He was very quickly convinced, however, that nothing short of a radical culture change was required. "It was very much a hospital model when it came to care. I remember the nurses in their headdresses going round. At 9.30 in the morning, I saw many men, and a few ladies, who had been moved out of the wards, with their curtained-off beds, so that the wards could be cleaned." He recalls having a "debate" about this that was the first step in the culture shift from treating patients to caring for residents.

"Since the old building had been deemed not fit for purpose, in addition to the day-to-day running, my role was to take the place forward." The complexity of simultaneously rebuilding, changing the way things were run and disposing of the mansion proved a considerable challenge and started to rule his life, says Gibson. He found he needed diplomacy. "The staff were absolutely committed but the overall approach had to change and none of us are good at the unknown. I had to encourage people to lead staff forward

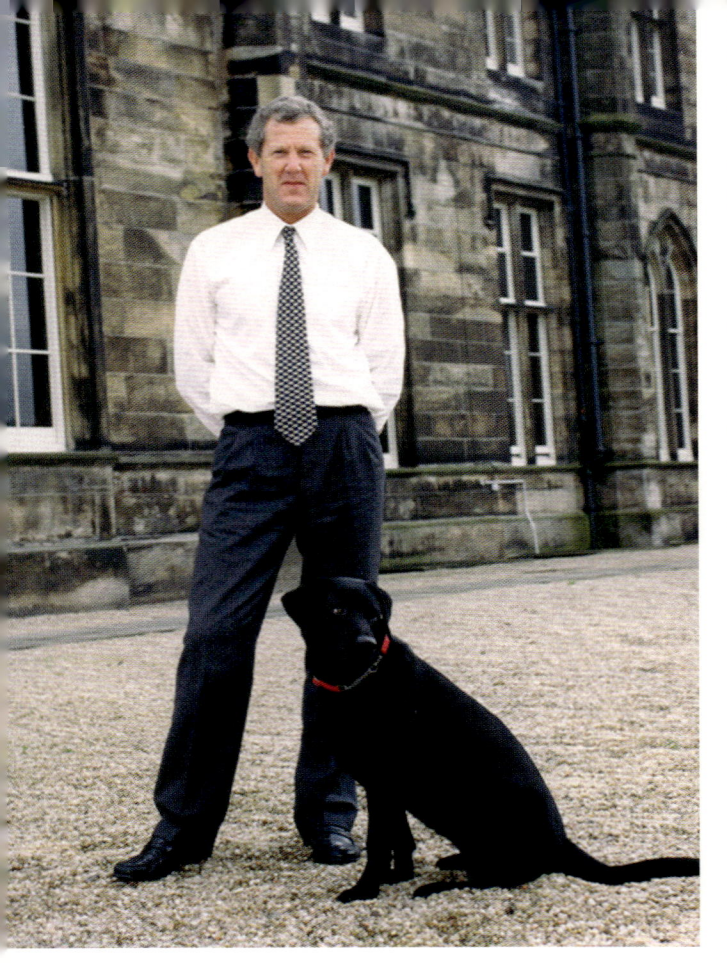

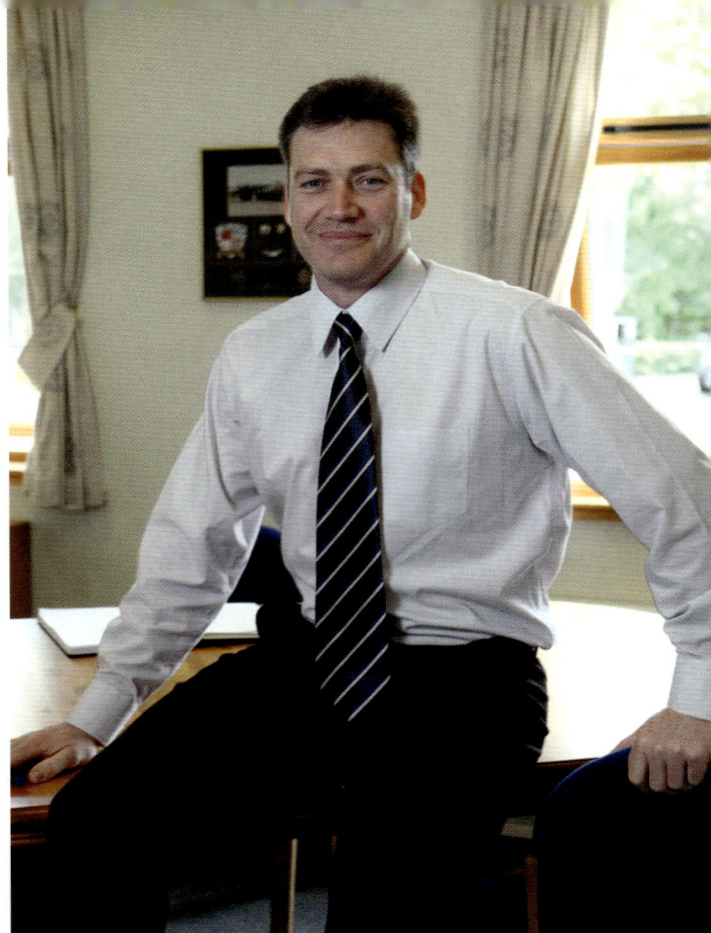

Above: Colonel Martin Gibson.

Above right: Major Jim Panton.

because care staff are very precious but we had to tell people who had been there for years that it was not as good as they thought."

Many care homes found it difficult to meet new requirements for fire safety and more privacy. Erskine, however, had to cater for the different needs of a wide variety of residents, whose ages then ranged from 30 to 99. He recalls they worked very hard with the regulators to meet the new requirements. Staff groups set up to consult on design resulted in rooms large enough take a hospital bed (a considerable plus as more residents need nursing) as well as a sitting area and en-suite.

There was also the difficult issue of funding and the wider one of how to publicise the change. "At the same time, we had to go through a rebranding exercise because we could no longer be the Princess Louise Scottish Hospital. It became Erskine after much discussion. If you are running a charity that is looking for tens of millions of pounds, branding is important. We were able to pay for all the new buildings and not run down the capital. The majority of people there now had nothing to do with combat but they were prepared to go to combat, so when you are fundraising you have to explain that to people when you are asking for their money. There were tough times but when you were having a bad day, if you went out and talked to people in the homes or the staff, you were inspired."

The workshops were an integral part of the Erskine formula from the beginning, with some of the early amputees involved in making artificial limbs for their comrades, perhaps the most practical demonstration ever of soldiers being brothers in arms. In Col Gibson's time the workshops included a printworks and a small furniture factory which provided sheltered employment for those unable to move back into their communities. There was also a nursery garden, growing produce for the kitchens and to sell to the public. All three eventually proved too uneconomic as the residents grew older and markets in these areas became increasingly competitive.

He acknowledges that Erskine was ahead of the curve with physiotherapy, speech therapy and recreation and an understanding that activities are very important to stimulate minds. He is particularly pleased that Erskine Park, the specialist home for people with dementia, has been very successful. "The staff have to have a close relationship and understand the whole person. I will always remember a Burns Supper where a patient who never spoke suddenly burst into song."

It fell to him to oversee what became known as "the great flitting" in 2000 to the new Erskine Home but the £20 million Erskine 2000 programme also included the establishment of Erskine Mains in the town itself, Erskine Edinburgh in 2001, the Erskine Park Home in 2006 and the Erskine Glasgow Home in 2007. There was considerable concern among some long-term residents about losing the companionship of the dormitory wards, in some cases after decades. Team spirit got them through. Gibson said he was always amazed at the resilience of many of the residents. "Despite illness, or injury from conflict, they have that spirit which is unique to people who've been in the armed forces, and that is what is at the heart of Erskine. It brings out the best in them. Even in adversity, there is an amazing sense of humour and it is our job to keep that going.

"The bottom line is that we are here to care for those men and women who put their lives on the line for their country, or were prepared to. Many of them had friends who made the ultimate sacrifice, and this is as true today as it was at the end of the Second World War."

Major Jim Panton, a former Apache helicopter pilot in the Army Air Corps who had previously led Poppy Scotland, joined Erskine as chief executive in 2009, leaving after two years to run his family's business in the Scottish Borders.

Lieutenant Colonel Steve Conway took the helm at Erskine at the end of 2011 after 26 years in the Royal Marines, followed by a stint overseeing emergency planning for NHS Scotland then taking on the task of chief executive of Orkney Health Board at a time of crisis. Seen together, this is a career path which forms a remarkably coherent preparation for running a healthcare charity for military veterans.

Many of the challenges he faces are similar to those of his predecessors. He has identified the key requirement as being able to move with the times and reflect people's changing expectations. With numbers in the British Army at their lowest since the Second World War, this means preparing for a reduction in the number of military veterans in the future. With recent conflicts in Iraq and Afghanistan and instability in the Middle East, there is a new public understanding of the dangers faced by the armed forces. Conway says: "We need to acknowledge there are service personnel today who need the same sort of care Erskine has provided since 1916 but they also need to be able to make the transformation to the civilian environment following their service career."

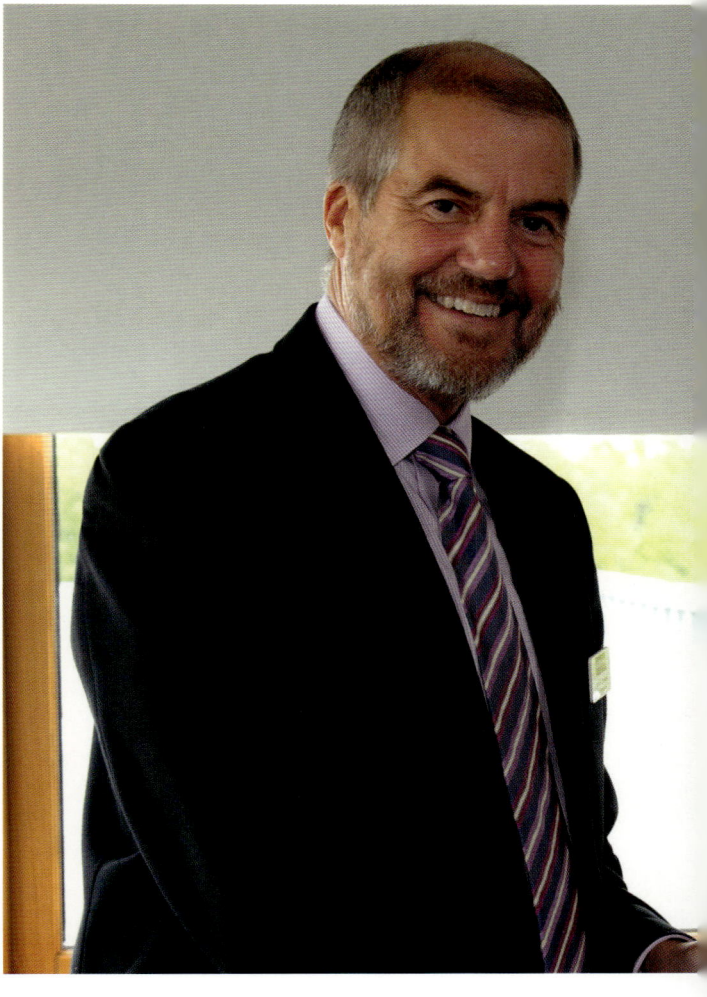

Lieutenant Colonel Steve Conway, current chief executive.

From Superintendent to Commandant to Chief Executive

Helen Bolland

"Sometimes the hardest thing is getting up in the morning, having a shower, doing your make-up and putting a smile on your face."

Helen Bolland contradicts the stereotypes of service veterans. She's young, female and appears to be healthy and fit when she greets visitors with a smile. In her neat cottage on the Erskine estate, there's a wheelchair folded discreetly next to her sofa and she occasionally uses the walls for support but the physical problems resulting from being catapulted from a Land Rover are the least of her difficulties.

Post-traumatic stress disorder (PTSD) is the umbrella term used to cover the range of debilitating symptoms, including flashbacks, nightmares leading to insomnia, paranoia and depression, which can be the lasting effects of being in terrifying situations witnessing the brutality of war. Return to routine after a traumatic experience can be particularly difficult for people with no obvious physical injury but who are just as disabled. Talking through exactly what happened is an important step in enabling the memories to be processed and stored safely. That was something Helen, as an intelligence analyst dealing with highly sensitive situations and bound by the Official Secrets Act, was unable to do.

Sport has become a key to keeping the horrors at bay. Cycling on a recumbent trike, swimming, archery, discus and shot putt are her chosen events and in 2015 she won three gold medals as a member of the British team in the US Air Force trials for the Warrior Games for injured and ill service personnel and veterans. That success has prompted her to consider a new challenge of taking part in triathlons involving cycling, swimming and wheelchair-racing.

Activities with other veterans are particularly helpful. As Helen says: "You don't need to tell service people what's wrong with you. They understand."

That's equally true of the challenges of day-to-day living. "The concept of Erskine is brilliant. My neighbours know I have my off days and the support is always there if you need it. It's also in a really good place. It's very peaceful, and that is vital, but is also fairly close to several hospitals and other facilities. The bustle and noise of cities is very stressful for people who are on automatic alert for sudden noises and the only loud bangs we have here are when there are fireworks for celebrations at Mar Hall hotel."

Originally from Prestwick, both her parents were in the army and, although they had both left before she was born, it seemed natural to her to join the army cadets as a teenager. Keen to see the world and gain a skill, she joined the RAF when she was 20. Her face lights up as she describes her job as an intelligence analyst and it's clear that she relished the challenge of learning difficult languages (Russian and Pashto, one of the languages of Afghanistan) as well as the highly responsible tasks of analysing interceptions in those languages, culling information from myriad sources, and briefing colleagues on what to expect before they went to Iraq or Afghanistan and passing on crucial information to forces in the field.

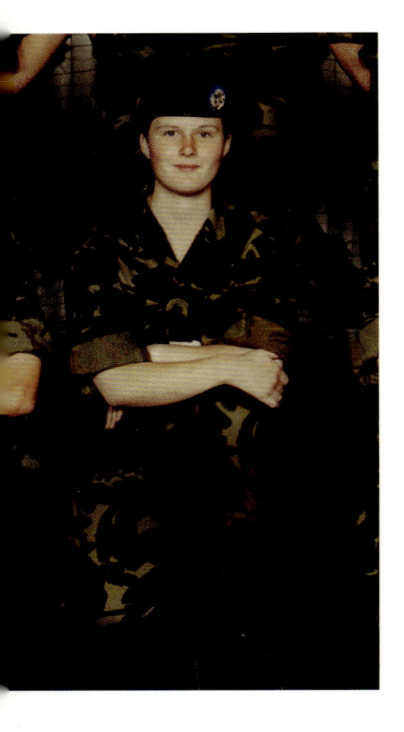

Helen in her army cadet uniform.

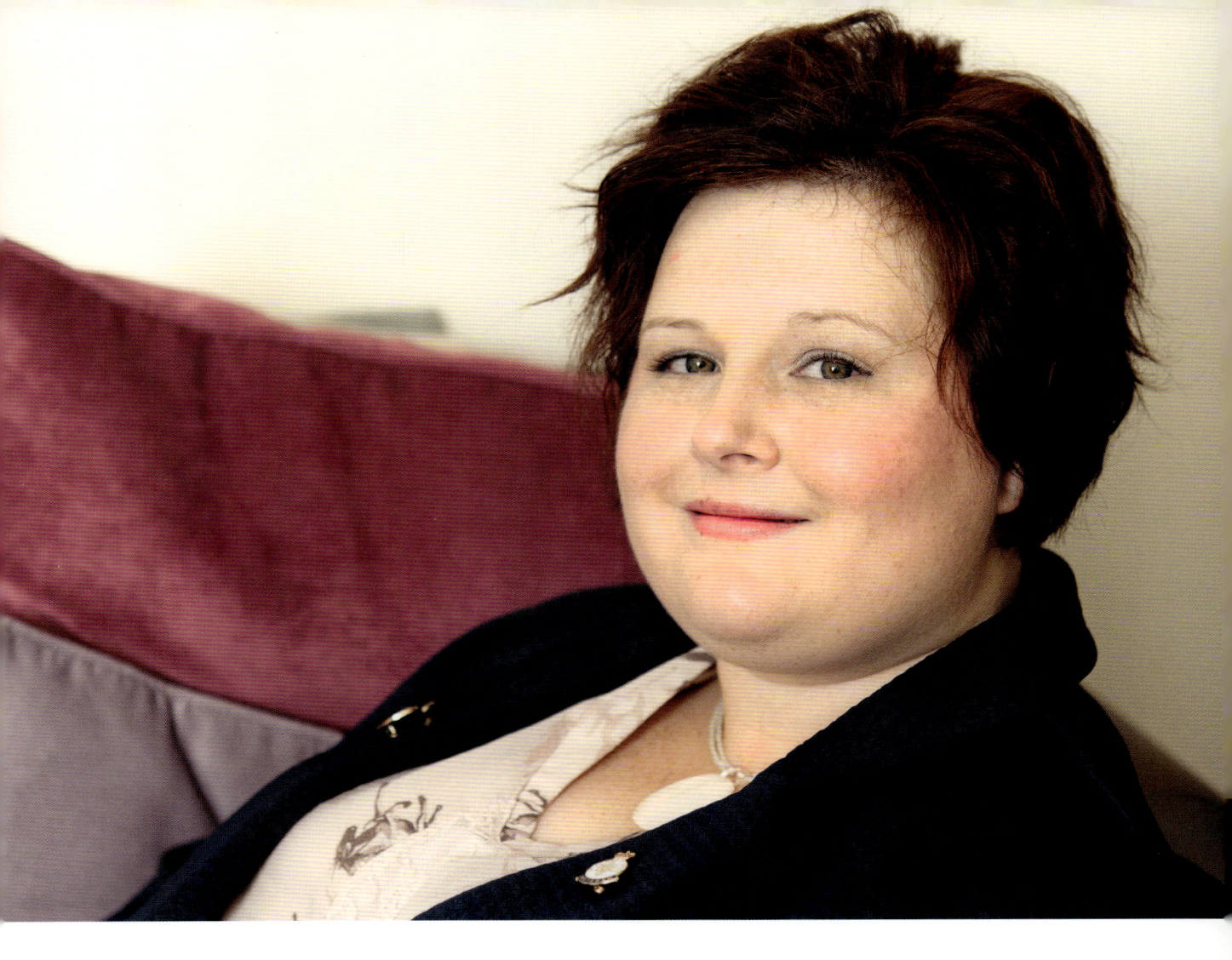

Helen Bolland, former RAF intelligence analyst, says: "The concept of Erskine is brilliant."

She found it fascinating, despite the very long nightshifts where nothing happened until the low ebb of 3am when suddenly a vital piece of information might appear. It's then that disastrous mistakes can be made. She recalls the example told to trainees of an analyst mishearing that a Russian regiment was moving to the strategic point in the very north of Russia bordering Alaska, where the then USSR met the USA. It seemed the Cold War was about to become red hot until a further check revealed the Russians were actually heading to the swimming baths.

"In the Iraq and Afghanistan campaigns we were feeding information about where the Taliban were in relation to the compound directly to troops so that they could get out without being seen because there was only one way in and out." She's incensed by the leaking of classified information about the US government's surveillance apparatus in 2013 by Edward Snowden. She believes the former CIA contractor will have put lives at risk: "He blew ongoing operations and made it easier for people like the Taliban to avoid ways of being traced."

Her seven years as an intelligence analyst included a six-month tour of duty in Iraq in 2005. In camp at Al Amarah in south-eastern Iraq (scene of an extraordinary battle in 2004, when British troops had used fixed bayonets for the first time since the Falklands War), they were attacked every night, including once when "a Chinese rocket came straight through where we were sitting and out the wall." Although she cannot reveal any details, what took

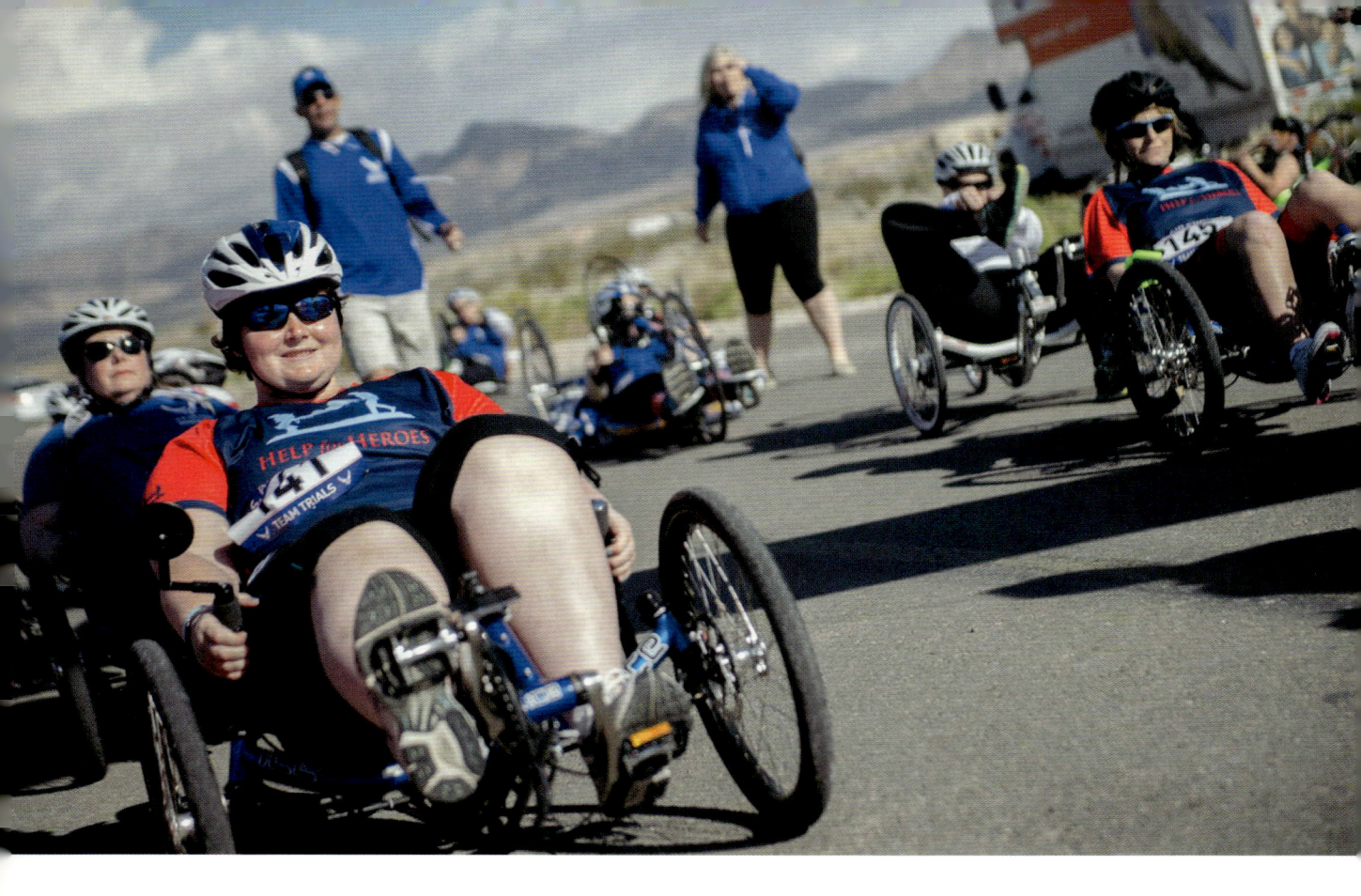

Competing on her recumbent bike, in trials for the Warrior Games.

the real toll was that even their best efforts could not always ensure complete safety for their comrades out on patrol.

She came home and started her Pashto course without having any leave. She then began to experience a variety of problems, which were diagnosed as PTSD only once she had been medically discharged in 2008. That was after considerable suffering. The first psychiatrist she saw simply said: "Pull your socks up, get your hair done, get a new dress and you'll be fine." This was a couple of years before the extent of PTSD among those deployed in Iraq was fully acknowledged but Helen also thinks that some service personnel felt there was a stigma attached to suffering from post-traumatic stress resulting in a reluctance to use the term. In her case the seriousness of her symptoms, which included depression, insomnia and paranoia, was not realised until she made a suicide attempt. Her difficulties were compounded by the fact that the nature of her job meant she could not discuss much of what had happened in Iraq with medical staff and she was no longer with colleagues from that time. It was assumed that the cause of her continuing symptoms was that she wanted to get out of the RAF. In fact her ambition was to gain promotion as an officer and sign up for 22 years' service.

Her eventual diagnosis came as a relief and reassurance that she was not going crazy but that her symptoms were caused by her experiences in Iraq. Nevertheless, discharge brought its own difficulties. Although there are resettlement courses, Helen was not well enough to go on one. She is still upset, years later, by the memory of being "pitched out" with no help or support at a time when "the hardest thing is getting up in the morning, having a shower, doing your make-up and putting a smile on your face." Since then, she acknowledges, the forces have "got their act together" for PTSD sufferers being discharged.

At 28, an age when she had expected to be independent, she had no idea where to go or what to do. Her parents had returned to Ayrshire after many years in England but she didn't want to burden them so, as a result of sticking a pin in the map, she went to Nottingham. She was not really fit to work and unable to find any employer who wanted her particular skills but took temporary, low-level jobs because she needed to pay the bills. It was a demoralising experience and to improve her employability, she studied occupational therapy. Once again, however, the PTSD forced her to give up after two years. The only realistic option was to move close to her parents in Girvan. Although it is an attractive seaside town, there were no work or social opportunities for a young adult in her circumstances and she did not fit into any of the priority groups for housing.

Yet, like so many residents at Erskine, Helen is extraordinarily determined. With a new aim of returning to university to study law and eventually provide advocacy for others, she undertook the access course at Glasgow University, despite that requiring a 180-mile round trip two nights a week.

It was clear she needed to be nearer more facilities and in 2014, at the age of 33, her life was turned around when she was able to move into one of the houses for injured forces personnel at Erskine. She wishes she could have done so far sooner but although she had always been aware of Erskine as a veterans' charity, she had never imagined it would be suitable for someone of her age until she read about the rebuilding of houses for veterans.

With the benefit of hindsight, she says firmly: "I think everyone who is discharged on medical grounds should have a social worker to match them with appropriate services." Gradually, she discovered some of those for herself, particularly groups set up specifically to help injured veterans. In 2013 she walked part of the Great Wall of China with the Band of Brothers, a group for ex-service personnel wounded or affected by conflict since 2001 and supported by the charity Help for Heroes. She recalls the seven days on the Wall itself as "really hard work, with steps varying in height from one inch to three feet and it was extremely hot" but was fascinated by the glimpses they had of the living conditions of the Chinese in the countryside far from Beijing. Most importantly, the new experience and focus on the physical effort combined with the camaraderie of the group helped her regain her sense of self. It also prompted her to take up other rehabilitation opportunities. These included spending a week learning horsemanship at Horseback UK in Aberdeenshire, set up by a former Royal Marine and staffed by veterans, to help wounded service members, particularly amputees and those suffering from PTSD, to rebuild their confidence and trust in others through gaining the trust of horses.

These positive steps have led Helen to take up her sporting challenges, despite loathing PE at school. It's significant that these have developed since her move to Erskine. It is now known that it is very difficult for symptoms of PTSD to improve when sufferers are exposed to stress and uncertainty. In essence, without some stability to build on, it is impossible to move on from the effects of the traumatic experience, for example, to allow both body and mind to step down from a permanent state of high alert. At Erskine the purpose-built housing in a peaceful setting with understanding neighbours provides the unique combination of independence and support that makes progress finally possible.

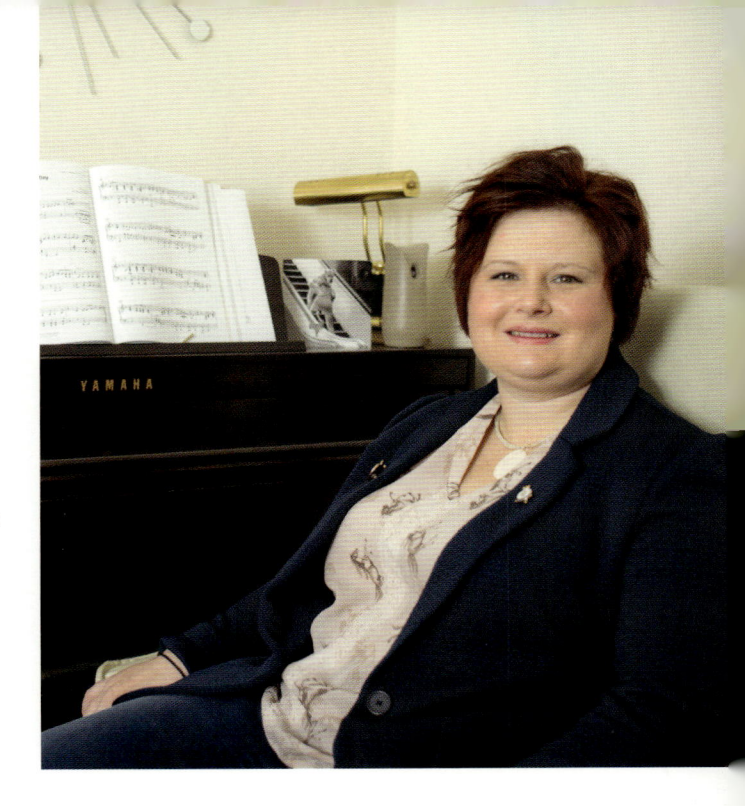

At home in her cottage at Erskine.

John Stonham

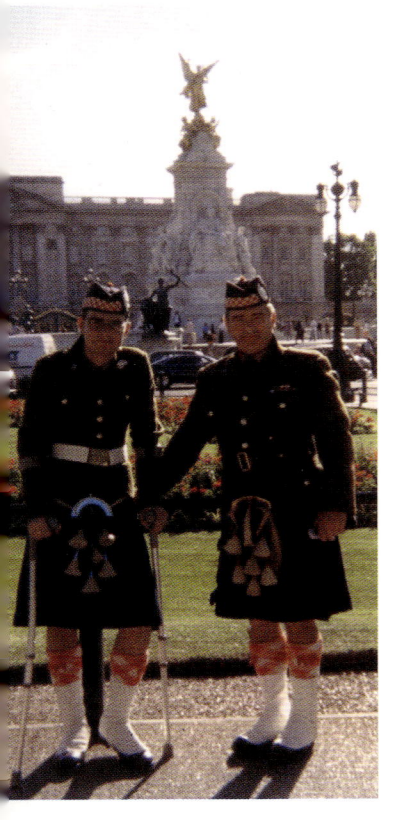

In uniform outside Buckingham Palace.

"I feel I owe it to the medics to live as good a life as possible."

Jobs were in short supply in Stranraer in the year 2000 when John Stonham was leaving school. Joining the army seemed the smartest move for a 16-year-old with drive and ambition but no immediate prospects. He joined the Argyll and Sutherland Highlanders and, after training, his first tour of duty was in Belfast. This was two years after the Good Friday Agreement but the fragile nature of the peace process was demonstrated in shocking fashion when the Holy Cross girls' primary school was the focus of violent sectarian hatred. Roman Catholic children and parents walking to the school through a Protestant enclave were threatened and spat at by Protestants following an eruption of violence among the youths in the area. The Argyll and Sutherland Highlanders were involved in protecting the young girls going to the school.

This was followed by a posting to Iraq in 2004. John was 19. He grins at the extent of his naivety, even after being shocked at what he'd seen in Belfast. As he says, he welcomed the idea of spending time in the sun. At the end of February, only 19 days after his battalion had arrived in Iraq, he was part of a patrol outside Basra, which had been sent to detain a suspicious tanker. He was providing "top cover" from the Land Rover, the most exposed position, and as they approached the tanker, it rammed their vehicle and he was thrown out sideways. The tanker then ran over his torso. He sustained horrific injuries, including fractures to his pelvis, a split thigh bone and a ruptured spleen and bladder.

"I remember seeing my foot stuck up in the air and thought I'd broken my leg. I kept falling asleep because they had injected my thigh with morphine and my mate was slapping my face and trying to keep me conscious. It took 40 minutes for the ambulance to come and take me to the field hospital. All I can remember of that is the padre reading the Bible to me because they thought I was going to die. They didn't have enough blood there because I was losing so much so they had to get extra from a US unit. By this time I was in a coma. I was flown back and taken to the John Radcliffe Hospital in Oxford. I woke up 19 days later and thought I had been shot in Belfast. I was very lucky to survive. I had 'died' four times because there was a blood clot in my lung."

The reality to which he'd woken was devastating because so much of his body had been crushed and broken. In addition, his damaged left leg had ballooned with toxins which were damaging his kidneys and required a major operation to save both the leg and the kidneys. Both were successful and, although the leg will never be what it was, he is profoundly grateful to be able to walk with a stick.

Before he got to that stage, however, there were 18 months of more operations and gradual recovery in hospital. Determined to be out of a wheelchair as soon as possible, learning to walk first involved a wheeled pulpit frame with high arm rests to enable him to stand upright, then a lower Zimmer frame. Once he could walk with two sticks, he was discharged from hospital. The physical milestone should have been matched by progress on the way back to normal life. That, however, proved to be an exceptionally bumpy road. John returned home to Stranraer but was unable to live with his family and the relationship with his girlfriend didn't survive the strain. He was allocated a flat in a block for homeless people, most of whom had additional problems such as drug or alcohol addiction and were keen to get their hands on his supply of painkillers.

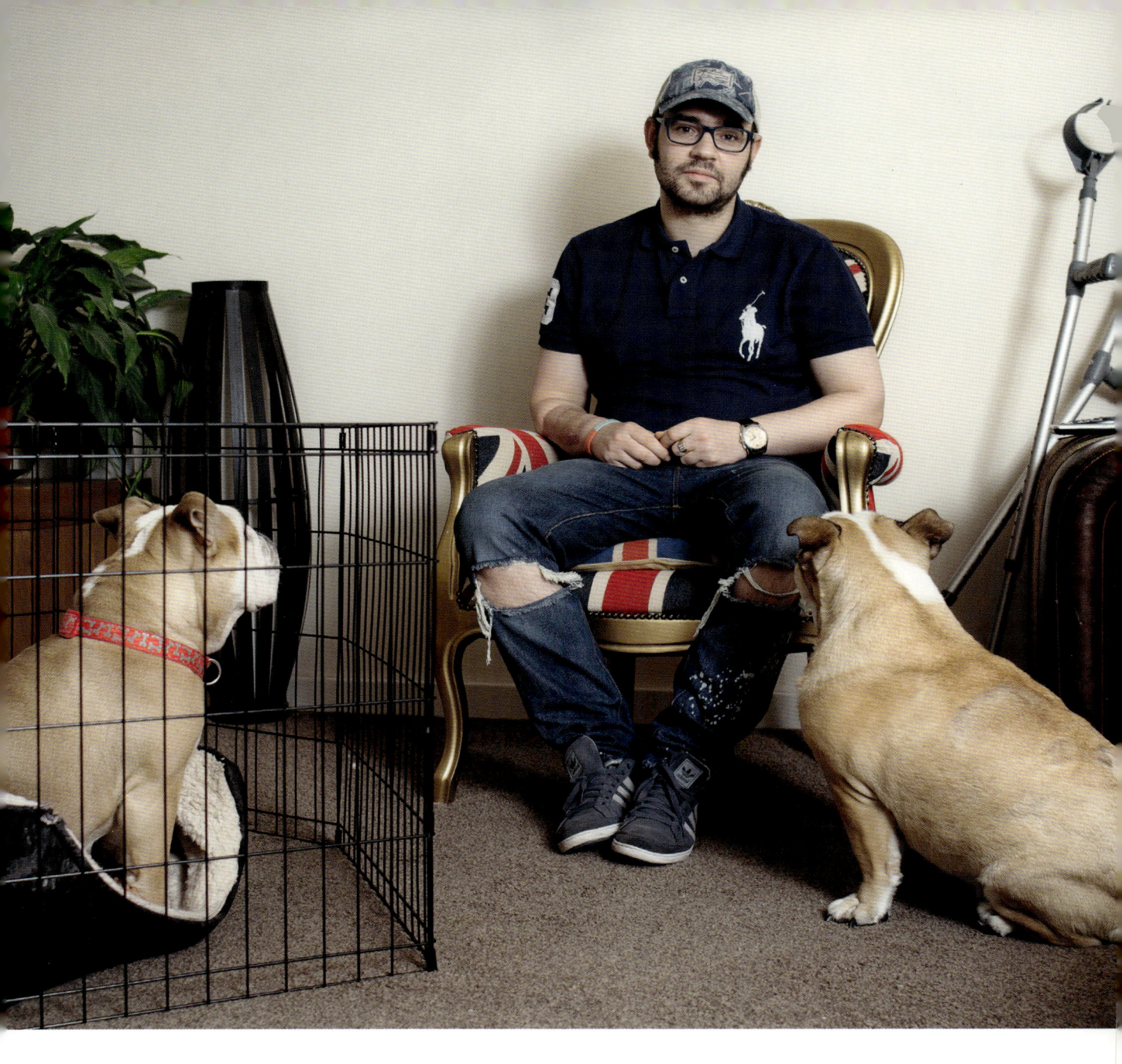

When the bins stored in an entrance to the building were set on fire, he had to be rescued bodily. Homeless, he was persuaded to tell his story to the press, which brought him to Erskine's attention. "I got a call from Erskine offering me two weeks' respite care. It was wonderful. They had no housing at the time but they said they would let me know when one became free. I wanted to move to Glasgow because I was attending hospitals there but there was no housing available, so I had to go back to homeless accommodation."

Life suddenly took a positive turn in 2006 when he was offered one of the Erskine veterans' cottages on the Bishopton estate. He no longer had to worry about his safety and

With bulldogs Lola and Bailey at Erskine.

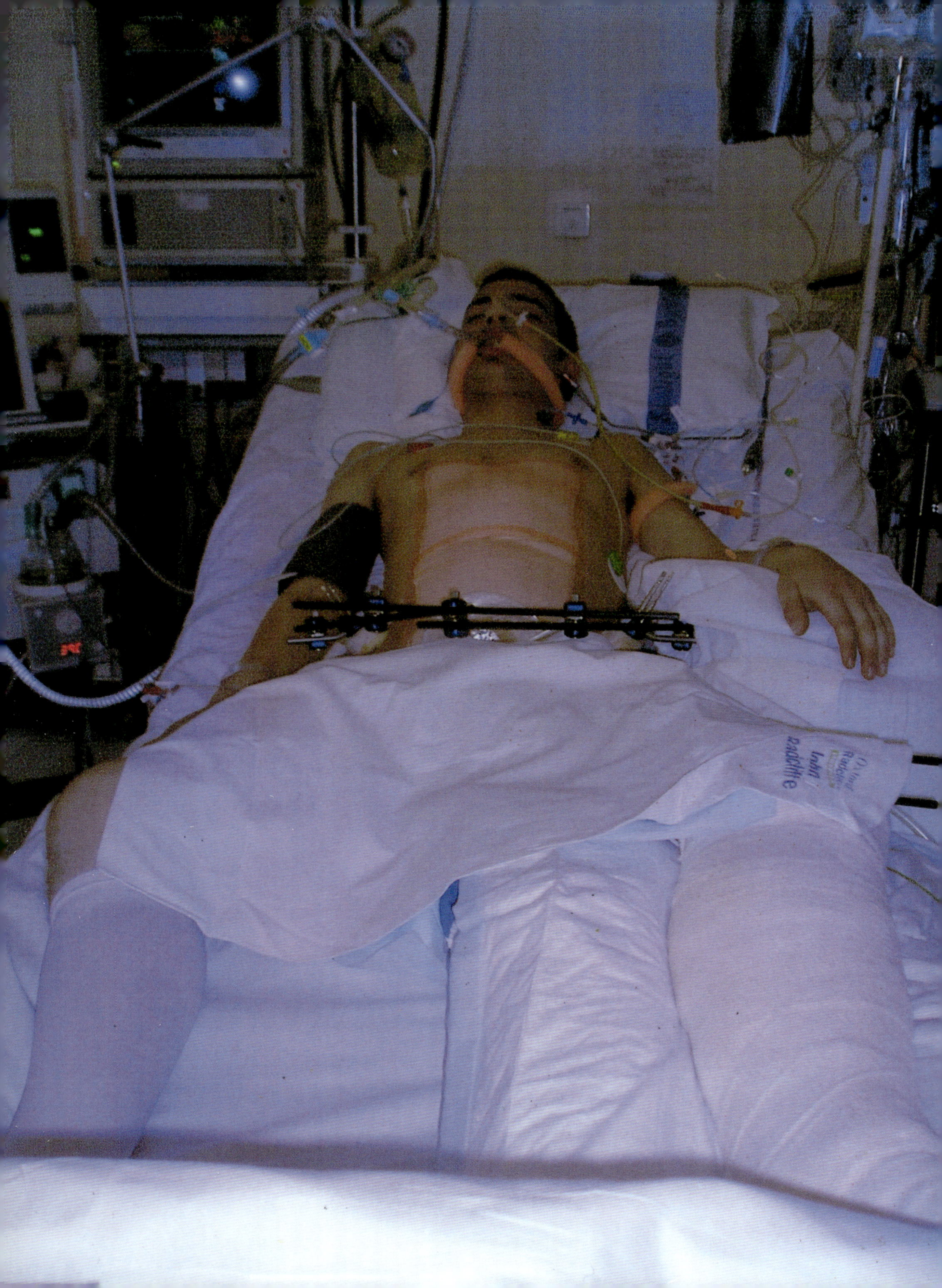

was able to have a pet dog to ensure he went out for walks. Bailey, named because she's the colour of the cream liqueur, is now getting elderly in bulldog terms and so he also has a young one, Lola, called after the Kinks' song. Still prone to puppy behaviour, she recently showed her disapproval of other bands by chewing the ticket for an Ocean Colour Scene concert. What happened next? John smiles broadly, pulls up the leg of his jeans to show the horrific evidence of his surgery and says: "Sometimes it pays to be a veteran." Of course they let him in with the remains of the ticket.

Why bulldogs? "I've always liked them. When I was growing up I liked watching wrestling and my favourite wrestler was known as the British Bulldog." At 31 and facing two more reconstruction operations, he's now acutely aware of the difficulties bulldogs suffer from having been bred to produce flat faces and in the future would like to provide a home for rescue dogs.

One step at a time, that future is taking shape. He's planning a trip to take in Iceland, inspired by the videos filmed in the homeland of another favourite band, Sigur Rós, Norway and Denmark. He's also considering volunteering to work with disabled children.

"I am lucky in that although I suffered from combat stress, I got some cognitive behaviour therapy from the veterans' mental health charity, Combat Stress. I don't know if that was because I was suing the army at the time and they wanted to show they were doing something for me. I'm now able to have a positive outlook."

Learning about the thousands of artificial limbs fitted to First World War veterans at Erskine has given him a new perspective on his own injuries and he quickly volunteers how humbled he has been by learning the stories of some of the Second World War veterans.

He does not say so but the difference between their experiences after demob and his are significant. As the scale of the wounded became known during the First World War, public dismay and a belief in the necessity of the war ensured Erskine House was transformed into the Princess Louise Hospital for Limbless Sailors and Soldiers and carried out its pioneering work on artificial limbs. The public was equally supportive of combat and grateful to those injured the Second World War. That has not been as true of recent conflicts with political division over UK involvement, particularly in Iraq. The National Health Service now provides medical and surgical treatment undreamed of in 1918 or 1945 but cannot provide the continuing care and rehabilitation built into the Erskine formula from the beginning.

Without that offer of respite care nine years ago, John's outlook could have been very bleak. His experience is mirrored by that of other veterans, particularly those who have been discharged on medical grounds, who have found great difficulty in fitting back into civilian life. Yet there are now many organisations which offer support, from regimental associations to the new charities like Combat Stress and Help for Heroes. It appears that what is missing is a strong link between the forces and the range of these services to ensure individuals who may need help are kept in contact. Erskine may yet have a new role to play in providing transition accommodation so that housing is one less thing to worry about while people are recovering their health and trying to find employment or permanent accommodation.

Erskine, says John, has been good to him. "They've protected me." He has also found friendship and has just been to the swimming pool with "my best mate who lives down the street."

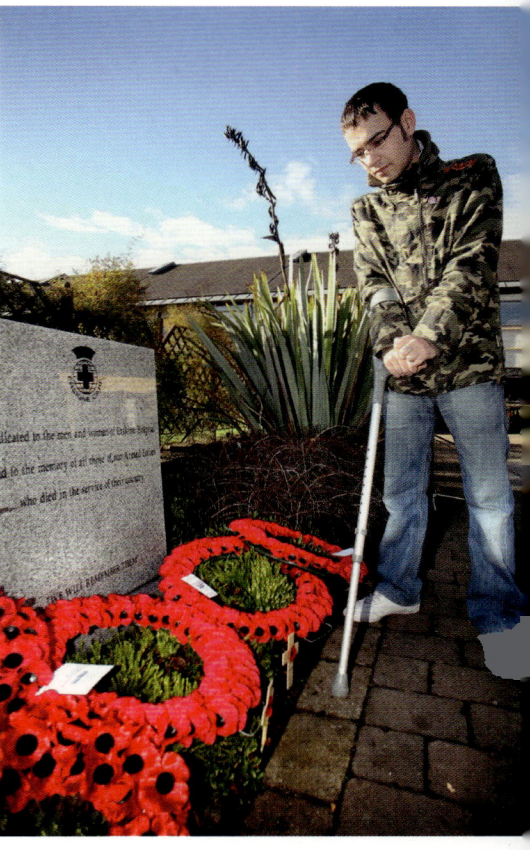

Above: Remembering fallen comrades.

Left: In hospital in Oxford after being airlifted from Iraq.

A New Century

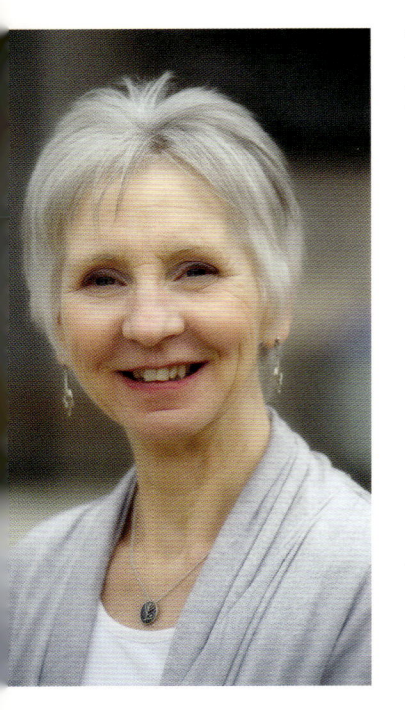

Erskine entered the 21st century with brand new, purpose-built homes designed to provide care for the elderly. It was the dawn of a new era but the challenge of balancing the books while providing the best possible standard of care is ever-present.

Sue Robinson, director of care, says: "We are privileged to care for often very vulnerable people."

The original concept of providing treatment and care for Scottish veterans remains the charity's central purpose but the old soldiers, sailors, airmen and the women who did their bit in the Second World War are now decades older than the men invalided home from the trenches from 1916. The residents range in age from mid-40s to 102, with the average 83. The homes at Bishopton and in Glasgow and Edinburgh offer 340 beds, with one-third designated for dementia and the rest for nursing care. In addition, Erskine now has partnership arrangements with care homes in Inverness, Aberdeen and Dundee to provide beds for ex-service personnel.

The military connection is seen as a core strength by chief executive, Steve Conway. "One of the key attractions to coming here is the camaraderie on which the armed forces survive. It is a help in difficult times and a lot of people want to maintain that. We do a lot of reminiscence and some of the performers who generously come to entertain the residents play wartime songs and that's very important for people with dementia."

Sue Robinson took up the baton of director of care at Erskine in 2011 from the NHS, where she held senior positions at the pre-devolution Scottish Health Department and Greater Glasgow Health Board. The move to Erskine in some ways has brought her career full circle because she trained as a nurse in the RAF (inspired by a recruiting advert in the cinema). She began her career as a midwife and district nurse in various parts of the country. It was as a district nurse that she first encountered the difficulty of looking after people with dementia, before moving into NHS management.

Because she believes the highest possible standards of care can only be achieved when there is a true understanding of the needs of the residents, all staff, not just nurses and carers, are given training in understanding the needs of the older people, and in particular those with dementia. "One of the domestic staff was asked to sort a pile of socks wearing gloves to simulate arthritic fingers and goggles to impair her vision, she eventually threw down the clothes saying she couldn't do it but she realised exactly how frustrated someone with these difficulties would feel." Some staff still lament the lack of camaraderie with the move from the large wards in Erskine House but exercises such as this are the modern equivalent of the young limbless soldiers' empathy for each other's difficulties. Sue Robinson recalls that the first time she arrived at Erskine, it felt different from all other care environments she had worked in. "The most obvious difference was the commitment of the staff. I've worked with some very good nurses but it was head and shoulders above anything I had ever come across in their interaction with the residents and their willingness to go that extra mile."

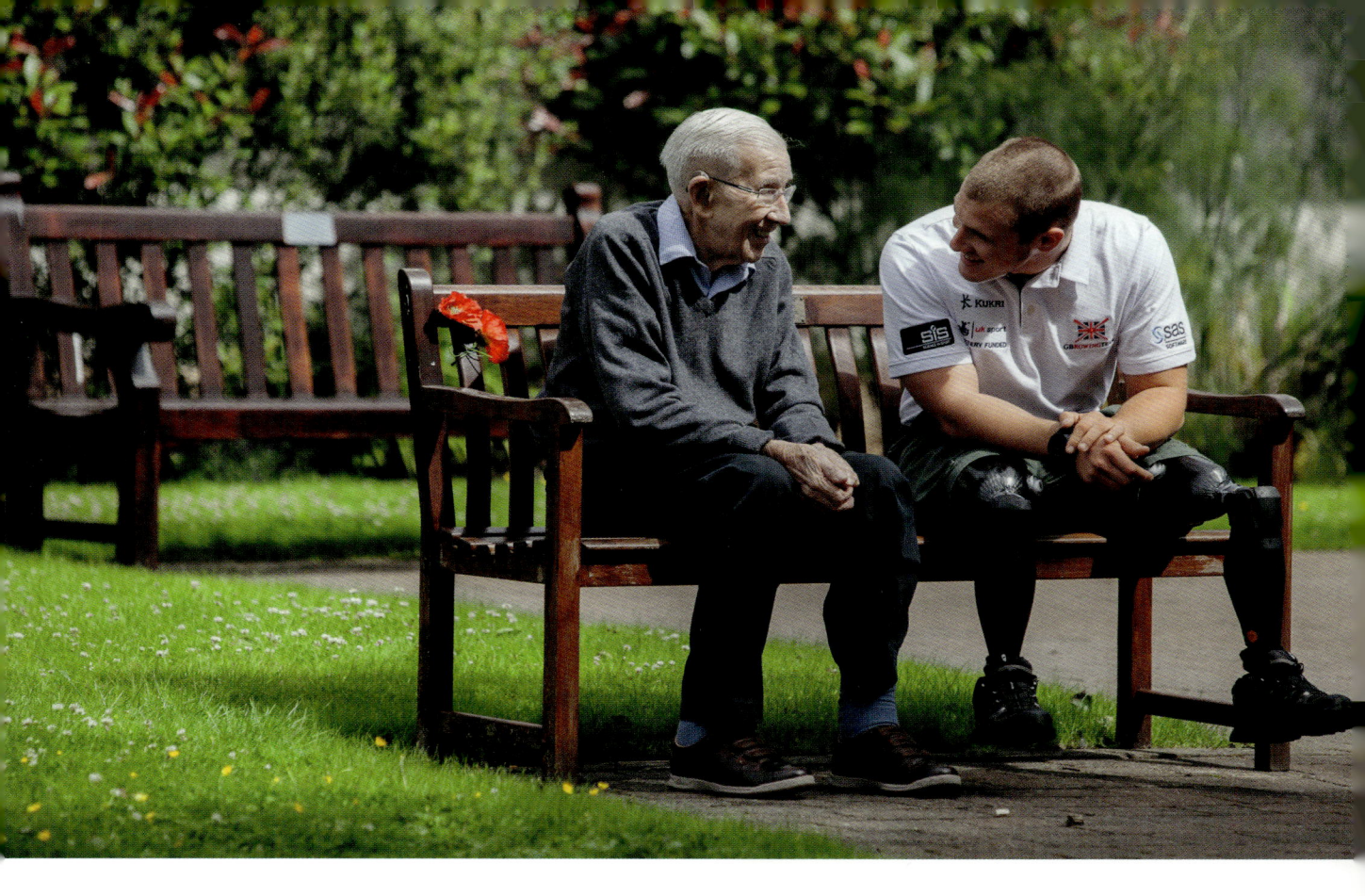

Veteran Donald Mathieson and Erskine Supporter Scott Meenagh.

The other difference is the common bond among the residents. Like many of those in her care, she finds her military background, brief though it was, provides a valuable point of connection. "Although we never forget that they are individuals, there is a common understanding among those who have served in the armed forces and it does seem to make a difference."

Equally important is attitude. Mrs Robinson explains: "I always impress on staff that we are privileged to be in a position where we are trusted to care for often very vulnerable people. The biggest tribute a family can pay us is to say that they trust us to care for their relative. We can never look after them in exactly the same way but we have to try and make it as good as we possibly can."

Although the buildings are now designed for purpose and staff increasingly well-trained in caring for older people, a new crisis is looming. Steve Conway is acutely aware that there will be far fewer ex-service personnel in the future and that Erskine will once again have to adapt to changing needs. "Part of my responsibility is to ensure that the organisation has a sustainable future and is able to meet the future need. I think we've got a challenge coming and this is not something you want to change quickly, but it is about trying to predict future demand and making sure we are ready," he says.

He expects to start focusing more on accommodation for the younger veterans as well as maintaining the elderly care. A start has already been made in that direction with elderly patients and staff from Erskine Mains being transferred to the main home at Bishopton towards the end of 2015. Consideration is being given to the future of the Erskine Mains site, with the potential to provide flats or build bespoke homes for independent living.

Erskine has a provided housing for veterans since the end of the Second World War and, following an extensive rebuilding programme, the 44 cottages on the estate are all less than

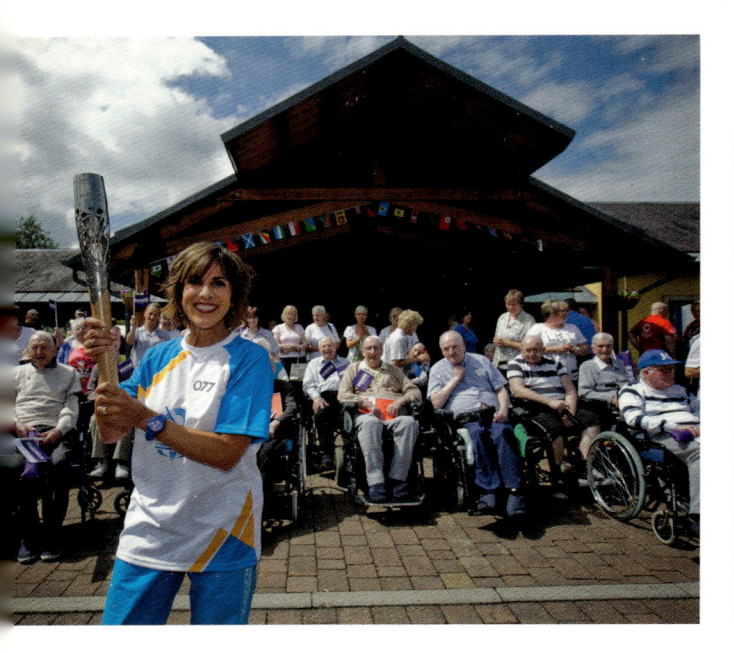

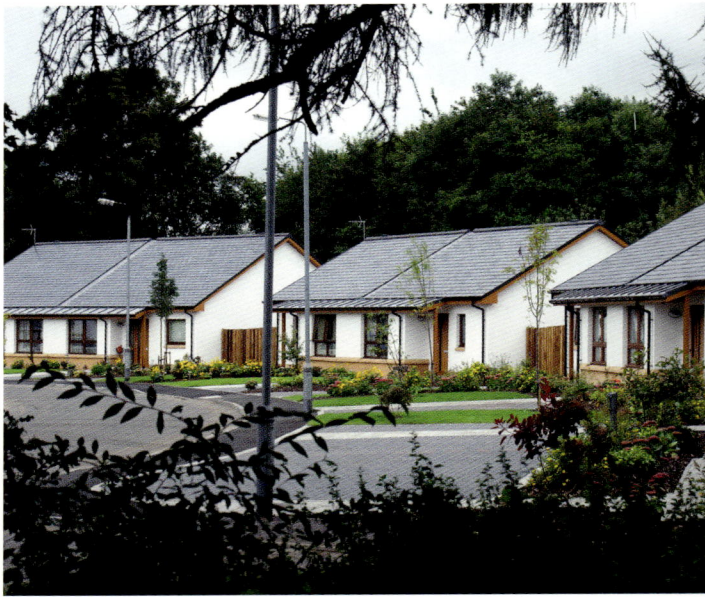

Above left: Shereen Nanjiani carries the Queen's Baton to Erskine en route to the Commonwealth Games in Glasgow in 2014.

Above right: The new veterans' cottages are energy-efficient.

10 years old. The original ones were demolished with one retained as a drop-in centre and a reminder of times past. The new-build was made possible by a particularly generous legacy, of just under £4m, which met over half the cost. Charitable trusts and foundations are increasingly keen to support capital projects rather than running costs. A recent example at Erskine was a grant of £500,000 from the Libor fund, which disburses the penalties paid by banks for rigging the inter-bank lending rate. This replaced all the lighting to meet the current standards which help people suffering from dementia, in particular, to see much more clearly,

Extremely welcome as these grants are, it can be more difficult to generate the steady flow of additional income to meet the running costs. The bulk of revenue comes from fees, with around one-third of residents funding themselves and the local authority paying for nursing care for eligible residents but this does not cover the physiotherapy, podiatry and speech therapy that make a great difference to many residents or additional services like hairdressing which add to the quality of life.

For Conway, this is where being a charity is hugely beneficial. "All of these things and the recreation teams in each of the homes, who provide activities for the residents seven days a week are only possible because we can raise charitable funds, otherwise the residents would have to pay extra. The other thing we are blessed with is volunteers, who make an awful lot of what we do possible, whether helping with activities, befriending residents." Just how blessed becomes clear with the statistics. There are just under 300 volunteers who together contribute 16,000 hours, the measure of just how well supported Erskine is by its local community, members of the armed forces and relatives of residents or former residents.

After seven decades of peace in Europe, the number of people eligible to come to Erskine will reduce considerably. Conway calculates that, based on the demographics, if nothing else changes, in 15 years' time we will need at least 100 fewer beds unless the eligibility criteria are changed. That has already happened. Today nearly one-third of the residents are women, among them a contingent of Second Word War veterans now in their 90s. They now include spouses of veterans as well as former forces members but they, too, appreciate the sense of camaraderie, particularly if they lived in married quarters. Some of the older residents who were demobbed in 1945 and lived completely different lives for many years but are keen to come back for care in their old age.

Laurence Binyon's 1914 lament for the fallen has been carved into memorials throughout the country and become familiar over decades of repetition.

They shall grow not old, as we that are left grow old:
Age shall not weary them, nor the years condemn.
At the going down of the sun and in the morning
We will remember them.

Yet it ignored those dreadfully injured by war, growing old and wearied not by age but by pain and frustration, condemned to struggle towards normality every morning, often unremembered. Good care for the elderly, particularly veterans, is an essential part of remembrance.

The other aspect of Erskine's provision is housing for veterans who need a supportive environment. "As long as there is a requirement for that we will continue to provide it," says Conway. "I think there will be a need for housing for younger veterans in the future. There is a housing need anyway so veterans fall into the same category. The attraction of sites like this and what some of the other charities do is they cluster housing for veterans which provides that community feeling. The vast majority of people make the transition. We are certainly looking at meeting housing needs whether its standalone housing as we have at the moment or flats or transition accommodation that someone might rent for us for six months, for example, while they find a job."

There was no expectation that in the 21st century a new generation of seriously maimed or traumatised service personnel would once again require the specialist services of a care centre for veterans. Thankfully, there are no longer thousands of young men having damaged limbs amputated but, tragically, there are still people losing legs to explosive devices. From the beginning, as well as mending broken bodies, Erskine helped to heal tortured minds. Long before the psychological wounds of war were called post-traumatic-stress disorder, and the understanding and fellowship of the military family was a vital component in rehabilitation. The cottages on the Bishopton estate continue to provide that supportive community.

The words which conclude the official record of the opening ceremony of 1917 could be seen as a challenge once all the amputees of the First World War had been supplied with Erskine limbs.

"Peace will long have been declared and a generation will have passed away before the purposes to which the stately building (Erskine House) has now been dedicated are fulfilled. But the Committee, to whom the great privilege has been afforded of acquiring permanently the house and grounds of Erskine and to whom a generous public, in money and kind, has given the means to maintain the house and grounds as a Hospital, feel sure that after the present purposes are served Erskine will take a foremost place among the great healing institutions of Scotland, of which Scotsmen are justly proud."

Despite a century of enormous change at every level from the personal to the global, the confidence of the founders of the Princess Louise Scottish Hospital for Limbless Sailors and Soldiers that its work would continue "after the present purposes are served" has been borne out in ways they could not have foreseen but which continue on a daily basis to demonstrate the best of man's humanity to man. May Erskine long continue as one of the great healing institutions of Scotland.

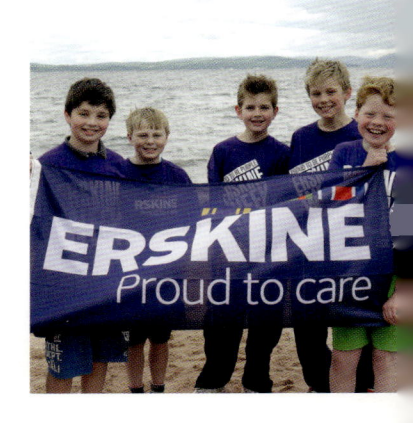

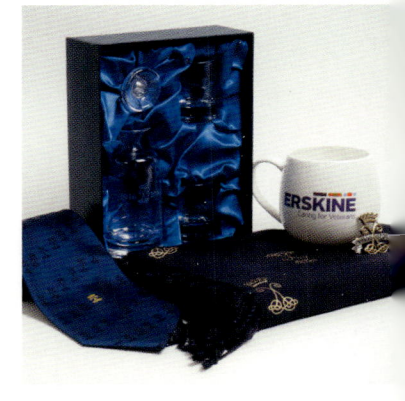

Top: Young supporters carry on the fundraising tradition.

Above: Products to mark Erskine's centenary celebrations include fine glassware, clothing and accessories.

Further reading

The Princess Louise Hospital for Limbless Sailors and Soldiers. Published by James MacLehose, 1917.

The Vanishing Willows, by John Calder. The Princess Louise Scottish Hospital, 1982.

Do You Sleep with that Leg On? by Harry Diamond. Erskine Hospital 2001.

Macewen of Glasgow – a Recollection of the Chief, by Charles Duguid. Oliver and Boyd 1957.

Lord Lister, by William Macewen. William Clowes 1912.

The Life and Teaching of Sir William Macewen – a chapter in the history of surgery, by AK Bowman. William Hodge, 1942

The Bletchley Girls: War, secrecy, love and loss: the women of Bletchley Park tell their story, by Tessa Dunlop. Hodder & Stoughton 2015.

Because It's Too Late, by Alex Lees; The Great Escaper: news report in The Herald, November 10, 2007.

Death of Roger Bushell – Love, Betrayal, Big X and the Great Escape, by Simon Pearson. Hodder & Stoughton

The Real Great Escape, by Guy Walters. Bantam Press.

Nuremberg: Evil on Trial, by James Owen (Headline Review); BBC report dated March 24, 2014: www.bbc.co.uk/news/uk-26706141

The Battle for the Falklands, by Max Hastings and Simon Jenkins. Pan.

602 Squadron. www.602squadronmuseum.org.uk

Stephen of Linthouse a shipbuilding memoir 1950–1983, by Alexander M M Stephen. Institution of Engineers & Shipbuilders in Scotland, 2015.

The Bringer of Hope, by William A Paterson 2014. Electronic copy available from Erskine.

The memorial garden, designed by Jayne Whitehead and rebuilt at Erskine 1914 by the Drystone Walling Association to mark the centenary of the outbreak of the First World War, poignantly recreates a garden abandoned to nature; its owner off to war.